Mapping Environmental Risk and Energy Communication

Environmental Communication and Nature: Conflict and Ecoculture in the Anthropocene

Series Editor: C. Vail Fletcher, University of Portland

This interdisciplinary book series seeks original proposals that examine environmental communication scholarship. In the Anthropocene era, the period during which human activity has become the dominant influence on climate and the environment, the need for highlighting and re-centering nature in our worldviews and policies is urgent, as collapsing ecosystems across the globe struggle to survive. Topics might include climate change, land use conflict, water rights, natural disasters, non-human animals, the culture of nature, ecotourism, wildlife management, human/nature relationships, food studies, sustainability, eco-pedagogy, mediated nature, eco-terrorism, environmental education, ecofeminism, international development, and environmental conflict. Ultimately, scholarship that addresses the general overarching question "how do individuals and societies make sense of and act against/within/out of nature?" is welcomed. This series is open to contributions from authors in environmental communication, environmental studies, media studies, rhetoric, political science, critical geography, critical/cultural studies, and other related fields. We also seek diverse and creative epistemological and methodological framings that might include ethnography, content analysis, narrative and/or rhetorical analysis, participant observation, and community-based participatory research, among others. Successful proposals will be accessible to a multidisciplinary audience.

Recent Titles in This Series

Mapping Environmental Risk and Energy Communication: Ecoculture in Energy Risk
By Barbara George

Conservation, Preservation, and Recreation at Glacier National Park: Navigating Tensions of Purpose in the National Park Service
By Maureen Wieland

Digital Worldbuilding and Ecological Readiness
By Cynthia Porter Rosenfeld

Mapping Environmental Risk and Energy Communication

Ecoculture in Energy Risk

Barbara George

LEXINGTON BOOKS
Lanham • Boulder • New York • London

Published by Lexington Books
An imprint of The Rowman & Littlefield Publishing Group, Inc.
4501 Forbes Boulevard, Suite 200, Lanham, Maryland 20706
www.rowman.com

86-90 Paul Street, London EC2A 4NE

British Library Cataloguing in Publication Information Available

Library of Congress Cataloging-in-Publication Data

ISBN 978-1-66692-648-4 (cloth: alk. paper)
ISBN 978-1-66692-649-1 (ebook)

∞™ The paper used in this publication meets the minimum requirements of American National Standard for Information Sciences—Permanence of Paper for Printed Library Materials, ANSI/NISO Z39.48-1992.

To family, friends, and loved ones who have spent time and cared about being in the environment—with me or on their own journeys. Here is to true hope for the future that we will care for and honor this earth.

Contents

Tables and Figures

FIGURES

TABLES

Introduction

There are powerful debates about how the rise of the Anthropocene has created deliberation about how energy is best produced and distributed in a world pressured by both the depletion of natural resources and global climate change. While some champion continued use of fossil fuels, an increasing number call for the implementation of alternative energy. Recently, technologies have enabled new systems of extracting energy like High Volume Hydraulic Fracturing (HVHF), complicating discussions of the future of fossil fuels or alternative energies. This complexity is particularly pointed in terms of infrastructure build-out such as pipelines and petrochemical plants as related to HVHF.

This book explores how citizens impacted by HVHF tell stories about environmental risks. The ability to access information to discuss environmental risks is socially situated. Deep ideologies linked to past activities—coal and industry—permeate areas like the Rust Belt and Appalachia and create "frames" that can encourage HVHF. Publics who envision banning HVHF or who would like to encourage a post-carbon future often find it difficult to use institutional tools or to find platforms to tell their stories in a meaningful way. This book explores how citizens impacted by HVHF tell stories about the conflict they experience in attempting to articulate environmental and human health risks. The book offers a case study of three communities in the United States: New York, Pennsylvania, and Ohio, each of which frames HVHF environmental and health risks differently based on different sociocultural histories. It is important to look at these case studies as these three states have widely different approaches to regulation; the cultural legacy of the "rust belt" in PA and Ohio makes current HVHF regulation particularly difficult. It is important to note, among these regions, the different locales mean that residents have various agency (or lack thereof) to define and act on environmental and health concerns. This book analyzes the communication patterns that institutions use for official risk assessments. Risk assessment communication often supports widespread fossil fuel infrastructure projects like HVHF.

Concerned citizens in Ohio and Pennsylvania, in particular, must navigate official and often complicated risk assessments that often steer users away from meaningful discussions about environmental risk, instead promoting pro-HVHF values such as economics. These "stories" are implicit or explicit in institutional risk assessments and often supersede other stories that embrace other values important to citizens, such as precautionary or environmental justice values that can be communicated in communities; this investigation of alternative possible communication patterns is also unique to this book.

This book uses an ecolinguistics and rhetorical lens to analyze the language that institutions use for official risk assessments. The International Ecolinguistics Association defines ecolinguistics as follows:

> Ecolinguistics explores the role of language in the life-sustaining interactions of humans, other species and the physical environment. The first aim is to develop linguistic theories which see humans not only as part of society, but also as part of the larger ecosystems that life depends on. The second aim is to show how linguistics can be used to address key ecological issues, from climate change and biodiversity loss to environmental justice.

Traditional linguistic analysis and critical discourse analysis, the latter of which analyzes "oppressive power systems," is a part of emerging ecolinguistics studies (Stibbe, 2015, p. 9). This book applies rhetorical and linguistic analysis to environmental risk processes; as Arran Stibbe notes, to "reveal the stories-we-live-by, opening them up to question and challenge them from an ecological perspective" (2015, p. 9). According to John Dryzek, a "discourse" is a "shared way of apprehending the world. Embedded in language, it enables those who subscribe to it to interpret bits of information and puts them together into coherent stories or accounts" (2005, p. 9). This book uses rhetorical and linguistic analysis to show how environmental risk language often supports widespread fossil fuel infrastructure projects like HVHF that become embedded in public policy.

My investigation also explores patterns by considering rhetoric or the "available means of persuasion" (Cox, 2006, p. 53), an important consideration in terms of how citizens use deliberative practices to navigate and participate in public deliberations about environmental risk and energy policy. I ground my work in notions of socially constructed rhetorics of risk as explored in the literature review, for example, Beverly Sauer's extension of traditional Aristotelian rhetorics to include both "postmodern and feminist awareness" (2003, p. 5) account for socially constructed notions of risk and those who are able to discuss risk at all. In Sauer's words, this means "that existing communication practices within industries are shaped and constrained by political and economic assumptions that may inadvertently silence or render invisible the kinds of information that decision-makers need to assess and manage risk in hazardous environments" (2003, p. 5). Additionally, Grabill and Simmon's "critical rhetoric of risk communication" (1998, p. 429) explores more deeply who is included in deliberations about risk communication beyond "experts" who simply disseminate information in a linear fashion to a passive lay person audience. In my research, I also found patterns of the rhetorical notion of stasis (Fahnestock and Secor, 1985) were helpful to categorize disparate policies in various states. Questions of fact (*is* there a risk?), questions of definition (*what* is the risk?), questions of value (is it *important to do something* about this risk?), and questions of jurisdiction (what exactly *ought* be done about the risk?) helped to clarify different approaches across states.

As noted earlier, concerned citizens in all states must navigate official and often complicated risk assessments that often steer them away from meaningful discussions about environmental risk, instead promoting pro-HVHF values such as economics. For example, the Environmental Protection Agency defines risk assessment as a process that "uses risk assessment to characterize the nature and magnitude of health risks to humans (e.g., residents, workers, recreational visitors) and ecological receptors (e.g., birds, fish, wildlife) from chemical contaminants and other stressors, that may be present in the environment" (2015), but there are questions about the language used in official risk assessments, particularly unknown risks inherent in a process like HVHF. Particular "stories" of risk are implicit or explicit in institutional risk assessments, and often supersede other stories that embrace other values important to citizens, such as precautionary or environmental justice values. Because New York considered human health, an environmental justice concern, as part of its state risk assessment, New York bans the controversial practice of HVHF drilling, while Pennsylvania and Ohio continue to allow HVHF drilling.

In considering rhetoric and ecolinguistics, this book also analyzes the language used by public participants who often identify as environmental activists to counter the pro-industry ideologies in public risk assessments. These "counter-public discourses" are used to change HVHF risk assessment in their local environments by offering discourses of environmental justice, precautionary and intersectional frames. This book includes an ecolinguistic and rhetorical analysis of various texts sponsored by environmental institutional regulatory governing bodies and, by contrast, applies ecolinguistics to understand new mental models about how to frame the environment. This includes texts sponsored by environmental activists, including screenshots of web pages, technical documents, maps (digital and paper), and public informational letters, and pamphlets.

ENERGY, ENVIRONMENTAL RISK, AND PUBLIC PARTICIPATION

The way in which conventional energy production and policy remain the status quo is noteworthy as emerging fossil-fuel-based practices are at odds with different ideological and discursive "frames" for future environmental policy and practice in response to environmental risks. Specifically, discourses might represent risks as linked to varied approaches to these energy policies and practices. Environmental risk, as defined by Whyte and Burton, is a "hazard or danger with adverse, probabilistic consequences for humans and the environment" (1981, p. 3). To understand environmental policy and environmental risk representation, one can look to scholarship that explores how the environment is constructed or framed by different people with different goals. How, for example, might those discussing "environmental risk" position themselves within, outside of, or as a part of the environment? The answer has important implications for how actors might construct policy about environmental risks (Killingsworth and Palmer, 1992; Hajer, 1995; Herndl and Brown, 1996; Myerson and Rydin, 1996; Dryzek, 2005; Cox, 2006; Lakoff, 2010). This book, which offers an ecolinguistics analysis of discourses surrounding hydraulic fracturing energy policy data from three key energy-producing states in the United States: Ohio, Pennsylvania, and New York, reveals different linguistic constructions[1] of environmental risks. These varied risk constructions lead to different energy policies, the consequences of which might be felt on local, state, national, and global scales. This study of language within varied socially constructed policies is salient in terms of the ways in which varied policy is often determined within different states. According to William Brady (2011), the positioning of state versus federal regulation of hydraulic fracturing leads to these varied representations of risks. "States are free to regulate hydraulic fracturing as they see fit, with the exception that state regulations must meet the minimum requirements of any applicable federal regulations" (p. 10). Of central interest in this book is how citizen participation in each of these states reveals discursive frames that promote different energy policies and practices. Because many oil and gas activities related to fracking are currently largely exempted from federal environmental oversight (Brady, 2011), citizens are placed in the position of navigating varied state and local participation mechanisms to represent risks related to this industry.

Michele Simmons (2007) explores definitions of "risk communication" and public participation, noting that the current definitional status of risk communication comes from a small group of researchers who tend to privilege the notion of risk communicators as "technical experts" who transmit risk knowledge to a broader public. Simmons' concern is that this assumption about risk communication does not "value the knowledge citizens can contribute to policy," resulting in a public that is largely marginalized during risk deliberations (p. 41). Simmons suggests definitions of "risk communication" that might encourage more "significant" citizen participation in environmental policy (p. 42). I include this more inclusive definition of risk communication.

The research in this book operates under the premise that public participation and deliberation about environmental risk can happen in many ways, from little or partial public involvement (typical) to full public participation (rare) (Simmons, 2007, p. 38–39). Later chapters examine the reading and writing citizens do in an attempt to influence environmental policy decisions to "access relevant information and make public comment to the agency that is responsible for a decision" (Cox, 2006, p. 84). The notion of an ideal space or procedure used to deliberate or reach public consensus about environmental risk is increasingly the subject of scholarly critique. The critiques attempt to build more complex and socially situated understandings of public participation and public deliberative spaces. Researchers question the way in which institutional sponsorship of deliberative spaces and procedures in addressing complex environmental issues has resulted in limited understandings of environmental risk and public participation (Szerszynski, 1996; Grabill, 2001; Bäckstrand, 2003; Simmons, 2007).

Regulatory risk reporting tools as texts and procedures that are sponsored by institutions to manage risk reporting. According to Jeffrey Grabill (2001) and Simmons (2007), powerful institutions support particular reporting tools and practices that determine how environmental risks are "defined, produced, distributed and consumed" (Simmons, 2007, p. 10).

This book uses the concept of risk reporting tools as detailed by Gene Rowe and Lynn Frewer, who referred to "environmental risk participatory mechanisms" as "processes, techniques, instruments" that enable citizens to participate in environmental risk deliberation" (p. 252). These might include public hearings, public surveys, or public written comment processes (Fiorino, 1990). These mechanisms might appear in online digital formats but at times might require a physical a presence at a meeting for public comment. These mechanisms increasingly fall under scrutiny by a variety of environmental communications scholars. For example, Rowe and Frewer (2005) call for more scholarship to attend to imprecise definitions of these mechanisms, uncertainties in execution of mechanisms, and lack of evaluation of these mechanisms.

As this book explores the way in which public stakeholders, public participants, and citizens can or cannot engage in public environmental risk deliberation as related to energy issues, it is important to unpack those terms the way in which those terms are used in research about environmental deliberation. The terms *stakeholders, public participants,* and *citizens* are often used interchangeably in research about environmental communication, but scholars do show some diversions in use. According to Mark Reed et al. (2009), *stakeholders* are those who are affected by decisions and actions, while Cox defines *stakeholders* in a more oppositional manner as "parties to a dispute who have a real and discernible interest (stake) in the outcome" (2006, p. 151), implying discord is implicit in environmental deliberation. Rowe and Frewer define *public participants* as actors who are involved in agenda-setting, decision-making, and policy-forming activities related to policy development (2004, p. 512). Similarly, Reed defines *public participation* as "a process where individuals, groups and organizations choose to take an active role in making decisions that affect them (Wandersman, 1981; Wilcox, 2003; Rowe et al., 2004)" (2008, p. 2418). Frank Fisher describes *citizen participants* as those involved in "deliberation on the pressing issue of concern to those affected by the decisions at issue" (2000, p. 32). By contrast, Thomas Dietz and Paul Stern's definition of *public participation* situates the participants as the *recipient* of institutional sponsorship:

> We are concerned with organized processes adopted by elected officials, government agencies, or other public- or private-sector organizations to engage the public in environmental assessment, planning, decision making, management, monitoring, and evaluation. (2008, p. 11)

In this book, it is important to be clear about these varied definitions as different perceptions of participants position actors toward particular courses of agency and action. Varied understandings of participant agency has consequences in the very real ways publics eventually engage and deliberate (if at all). Understanding assumptions about what a stakeholder, public participant, or citizen "is" becomes embedded in the very tools the participants in my book use to attempt environmental deliberation. For the purposes of this book, stakeholders, public participants, and citizens are actors who deliberate in any way about environmental issues that might impact them.

ECOLINGUISTICS: STORYLINES, FRAMES, AND IDEOLOGIES: RHETORICAL APPROACHES TO RISK (IS/ OUGHT)

Ecolingustics help to understand how public participants can deliberate about risks. To do so, it is important that the way stakeholders think of risk is related to "stories" that they believe about the environment, which informs their discourse. Dryzek (2005) points to the importance of analyzing language within environmental discourse: "this inquiry (environmental discourse) rests on the contention that language matters, that the way we construct, interpret, discuss, and analyze environmental problems has all kinds of consequences" (p. 10), particularly in terms of contested "deliberations" about environmental risk that result in policy or framework maintains agency in policy or practice. Similarly, environmental discourse scholars Hajer and Versteeg (2005) refer to social constructions of language and context, most notably in terms of the limits language can place on the possibility of participating in a given social activity. This understanding of environmental discourse relates to Critical Discourse Analysis's inquisition into the ways in which language frames who has power in given social constructs: "Language is not a neutral messenger of given interests and preferences, but it influences their very formation. Moreover, it enables and limits the range of practices and interactions in which actors can engage" (p. 166). In particular, Hajer and Versteeg cite the importance of discourse scholarship in investigating the "complex interactions" of environmental policy-making as related to risk: "Concepts, such as sustainable development or the precautionary principle, are not and simply cannot be imposed in a top-down way, but are continually contested in a struggle about their meaning, interpretation and implementation" (2005, p. 176). Hajer and Versteeg show that discourse analysis reveals facets of deliberation: "In trying to make sense of this struggle, discourse analysis has three particular strengths: the capacity to reveal the role of language in politics, to reveal the embeddedness of language in practice and to illuminate mechanisms and answer "how questions" (2005, p. 176). Similarly, Hajer suggests that understanding the institutional contexts in which words are produced and circulated helps us to understand the socially constructed nature of discourse:

> developments in environmental politics critically depend on the specific social construction of environmental problems. We do not simply analyse what is being said, but also include the institutional context in which this is done and which co-determines what can be said meaningfully. (1995, p. 5)

Ecolinguistics can then point to ways that our minds "frame" human perception of the environment. Ecolinguistics are a part of a broader understanding of sociolinguistics or understanding how language and culture influence each other. George Lakoff refers to framing as unconscious schemas which include "semantic roles, relations between roles, and relations to other frames" (2010, p. 71). Additionally, these frames move beyond an individual, they are often shared as cultural viewpoints that "inform the practices of a community of social organizations" (Brulle, 2010, p. 2). Dryzek argues that these "frames" inform ideologies or shared positions and perspectives about the environment and the construction of environmental issues (2005). For example, Stibbe (2015) points to the ways in which "development" frames often hamper environmental discourse (p. 54).

This book explores ideological frames by pointing to empirical study examples of discourse legitimation patterns, metaphors, and erasures existing within texts and procedures in which public participants engage when attempting to represent environmental risks associated with high-volume hydraulic fracturing (HVHF) or fracking in their local communities. These frames are rhetorical in nature; the pull of the Is/Ought in terms of public policy is predicated upon the ideologies from which they spring. The book also reveals ways local, state, and federal environmental institutions in New York, Pennsylvania, and Ohio frame the "environmental risks" of HVHF, and how participants respond to those representations. Through this, one can analyze specific environmental policy discourse frames, or specific ways of understanding the world through language, and the ways in which those discourse frames shape environmental risk deliberation and policy.

John Dryzek (2005) suggests different environmental discourses are ideological in that "discourses construct meanings and relationships, helping to define common sense and legitimate knowledge" (p. 9). Similarly, Arran Stibbe (2015) defines environmental ideologies as "belief systems about how the world was, is, will be or should be which are shared by members of particular groups in society" (p. 23)—he extends this to the notion of metaphors and erasures. These various discourses rest on assumptions that allow for shared understandings of a particular discourse. This book analyzes discourses, or storylines, that have underlying assumptions about emerging energy policy, or rhetorical consideration of "Is/Ought" as related to environmental risk, as can be seen by pointing to examples of discourse legitimation patterns, metaphors, and erasures.

For example, to address the way in which consent for HVHF happens linguistically, linguistic scholarship more clearly theorizes the "legitimation" of power found in texts or mechanisms navigated by participants. Discourse structures position information that directs users to normative conclusions about content in texts (van Dijk, 2003, p. 358; van Leeuwen, 2007, p. 92). In chapter 2, this book shows how pro-industry storylines "frame" particular ideologies through language. Language normalizes particular behaviors, often within institutional risk reporting tools given to public participants that result in the rhetorical "ought" of a particular policy. Frank Fischer (2000), an environmental communications scholar, explicates how the framing of neopositivist strategies used by chosen experts empowers and creates legitimacy for experts and disempowers public deliberation opportunities about contested environmental claims:

> Because of the fundamental differences in the legitimacy and power of their respective languages—technical vs. everyday language—the interaction between the technocratic planners and the members of the local community tends to give shape to an unequal communicative relationship . . . Such characterizations capture a belief in the superiority of scientific policy methods over political decision processes. (p. 18)

DESTRUCTIVE DISCOURSES

Environmental discourse scholars and ecolinguists point to problematic relationships between discourses and the environment. For example, Dryzek (2005) reveals concerns about an environmental "managerial" discourse approach, and Stibbe explains troubling issues of "economics discourses" (2015, p. 24). Stibbe refers to these as "destructive discourses" "[that are] considered to play a role in ecological destruction, and are highly widespread" (2014, p. 24). In chapter 2, this book analyzes the legitimization of storylines of managerial and economic discourse approaches is largely applied to permitting *for* HVHF activity. Examples in chapter 2 show how language shapes public participant's orientations toward any deliberation about HVHF. The Ohio Department of Natural Resources (ODNR), the state agency participants expect to regulate HVHF activity, overwhelmingly represents nature as a resource—something that ultimately can be managed for profit. According to Ohio participants, institutions adopt attitudes that place a value on the management of resources to capitalize on profits. The legitimation of this pro-industry ideology occurs through the use and normalization of language frames that position the HVHF industry as "legitimate" though HVHF risk often had yet to be defined, tested, and regulated.

Capitalist discourse frames might frame environmental risk very differently than other discursive frames. Environmental discourse scholars contend that current energy policies in the United States are positioned to legitimize "development" or "industry" frames (Dryzek, 2005). In the industry frame, environmental risks emerge and are dealt with in response to inevitable industry development. This is in opposition to a precautionary frame, which urges caution in terms of what an industry can or should do. Similarly, environmental discourse scholar Harvey explores the notion of a "standard view" of environmental policy as a type of "environmental management," which ultimately supports existing extractive and production practices promoting "business as usual" capitalist economic systems (1999).

Concerns of power and agency and environmental risk are compounded by unequal access to risk reporting tools and the ways these tools are used by different agents. Of particular concern in this book, then, are moments when discursively constructed literacy practices tend to guide a premeditated outcome, one that stymies alternative discussions, such as renewable energy development, or does not represent, fully, risks inherent in unconventional fossil fuel production. In chapter 2, destructive discourses are analyzed through Dryzek and Stibbe's notion of linguistic environmental "metaphors" and through Stibbe's notion of "erasure," both of which have strong links to powerful ideologies that frame the way particular stories are told.

POSITIVE AND BENEFICIAL DISCOURSES

However, competing discourse frames can challenge what Simmons terms as "pseudoparticipation" of citizens in deliberations about environmental policy (2007, p. 38) that "normalize" an "inevitable" future as framed by dominant discourses (Hajer, 1995; Dryzek, 2005). These can be considered to be "positive" or "beneficial" discourses (Martin, 2004; Stibbe, 2015). Environmental justice frameworks, for example, challenge "industry" or "standard" ideologies due to a concern with "the legacy of a disproportionate burden imposed on poor and minority communities by environmental harmful conditions, [and calls for] more inclusive opportunities for those who are most affected to be heard in the decisions made by public agencies" (Cox, 2006, p. 290). Other scholarship reveals calls for understanding complexities involved with representing environmental risks, so there are possibilities for publics to find meaningful spaces to deliberate about these risks, revealing a different rhetorical "is/ and ought" that can result in a different policy consideration. This book reveals how complexities inherent in energy discourses are often used to highlight the practice of fossil fuel energy extraction while obscuring energy alternatives. Many environmental deliberations involve concepts of risk, or an acknowledgment that particular actions might be disruptive to human, animal, or plant ecologies. These deliberations also consider uncertainty, or the acknowledgment of "unknowns" in terms of how complex socio-ecological systems might react or interact.

As such, it is important to understand the rationale for my use of ideological frames of "precautionary" and "environmental justice" within studies of environmental risk representation. While environmental laws ensure citizens' legal right to know, right to comment, and right of standing (legal status) about an environmental risk issue that might impact them (Cox, 2006), there are questions about how public participants read and write to navigate these processes and documents. The discourses informing participatory mechanisms and risk reporting tools are of central concern and analysis in this book because they frame affordances or constraints for participants. Simmons is particularly concerned about constraints, or the way in which citizens wanting to contribute are part of "unequal power relations that currently work to marginalize public involvement" (2007, p. 4). Simmons' analysis is central in understanding how public participants might choose to engage with, subvert, or work beyond existing regulatory risk reporting tools. To attend to Simmons' concerns, this book analyzes "precautionary" and "environmental justice" risk scholarship and highlights the analysis of primary data of participants' use of alternative frameworks to understand HVHF risk.

Chapters 3 and 4 include an analysis of precautionary discourse within Dryzek's "green" storyline—these can be thought of as intervening in the status quo. Precautionary perspectives recommend that when industrial activities might be associated with environmental risk, precautions should be taken so the burden of proof falls not on the public but on the proponent of the industrial activity (Steingraber, 1997, p. 284). Precautionary risk reporting is designed to promote proactive rather than reactive policies and has the potential to offer new possibilities for stakeholders to contribute to environmental risk analysis (Whiteside, 2006). This book offers an empirical study to detail ways in which participants employ precautionary perspectives to monitor HVHF risk by analyzing what Stibbe refers to as "salience" and "re-minding" in discourse. Salience, according to Stibbe, is "a story in people's minds that an area of life is important or worthy of attention" (2015, p. 162). Re-minding is "explicitly calling attention to the erasure of an important area of life in a particular text or context" (Stibbe, 2015, p. 162). Precautionary discourses show examples of both—that uncertain futures of public participants are worth discussing, and that this discussion has largely been erased in risk discussions.

Public participants in this book also pointed to environmental justice concerns in their effort to represent or report environmental risk as related to HVHF. Chapters 3 and 4 refer to environmental justice discourses. Environmental justice is the acknowledgment of the unequal distribution of environmental risks like toxins (Bullard, 1993). Within environmental justice discourse, notions of "intersectionality" help stakeholders to consider ways stakeholders living in HVHF areas that might be impacted by multiple risk factors. Wendy Smooth refers to Crenshaw's notion of intersectionality as a tool that might "make sense of the experiences of people who find themselves living at the intersections of social identities . . . concerned with systems that give meaning to the categories of race, gender, class, sexual identity among others" (2013, p. 12).

Environmental justice discourse allows for stakeholders to discuss the collateral effects of manufacturing, disposal, and transport of natural gas via the HVHF industry, which occurs in all three states, resulting in varied and complex representations of "risks" related to HVHF regulation among and even within states that highlight "systems of oppression that maintain power hierarchies" (Smooth, 2013, p.11). Scholarship about intersectionality showcases the ways in which complex concerns might be articulated to challenge normate views about public participation and policy planning, allowing for expanded definitions of who might be included in "public" participation as related to environmental risks, expanding notions of agency beyond industry or governmental leaders (May, 2015; Woehrle, 2014). Scholars exploring intersectionality suggest that risk deliberation must take into account overlapping "risks" within energy extraction. Environmental justice scholars explore expanded notions of how citizens might contribute to environmental risk reporting by understanding justice in several arenas: distributive economics, toxins and pollution distribution in space, and toxin and pollution risks through time (Holifield, Porter, and Walker, 2010; Walker, 2010; Nixon, 2011). Examples in this book specifically highlight instances of intersectional concerns as defined by participants that are often missed by institutional environmental risk participatory mechanisms, again by analyzing "salience" and "re-minding" in environmental risk discourse. I offer a green politics discourse analysis in chapters 3 and 4.

PARTICIPANT SELECTION

This book explores the experiences of research participants who self-identified as fracking activists. These participants encourage, in a critical approach to energy risk assessment and a wider discussion about post-carbon futures that rejects the "inevitable" future of HFHV as an energy resource and considers renewable energy options. I explore the notion of "identity" in terms of participant/activist identity positions because participants navigate existing regulatory risk reporting tools based on what they perceive their relationship with the environment to be. As noted earlier in the chapter, Stibbe (2017) theorizes the ways in which human behavior is predicated upon both social and self-identities. Stibbe discusses the ways in which actors who accept a particular identity tend to "conform to the mental model of what that kind of person says and does" (p. 107). What I found to be telling were the ways in which individuals shifted identities toward "activism" in order to, as Stibbe theorizes, "behave in ways which help protect the systems that life depends on" (p. 107). This book explores how activists seek to expose risks of fossil fuel technologies and the literate practices that highlight deliberations that allow for alternatives to fossil fuels. For example, activists reported patterns of dissatisfaction in the way in which renewable energy discursive frames and sources are discouraged, implicitly or explicitly, in institutional environmental risk communication. Several activist participants from each state who have shared literate artifacts[2] at public meetings or in a public setting (activist websites).

Many participants in my study identified as activists in our interview/think-aloud protocol sessions, but all did not necessarily share that identity position with local neighbors or even extended families. Some feared public or industry repercussions or feared being misunderstood or labeled as radicals. Some identified as activists only in so much as they felt that they had attempted to use "traditional" environmental risk reporting mechanisms, but when those failed, they had to seek alternative literacies, and, at times, they were required to invent literacies. These participants were very concerned that they not be seen as activists or "radical" in a public manner at all (though they identified as activists for the purposes of my study with the agreement that they be studied anonymously). Instead, they felt that institutional mechanisms should more directly serve publics concerned about environmental issues. In the case of New York, "fractivist" identities are particularly interesting—as some policies (banning of HVHF) have since been instituted since December of 2014, but not others (transport and storage of unconventional oil and gas).

Other participants were comfortable with the identity of or even self-identified as "fracktivists" or environmental "radicals," noting they believed that they were defined by state and federal institutions as "radical" simply because of their opposition to the industrial HVHF. Many of these participants, including those who assumed an identity as a "radical," critiqued the notion of the identity of "radical" imposed on anyone who might question institutional "framing" of relationships between humans and the environment. Several, but not all, participants had been arrested for protesting fracking activities; the protests were all in the form of positioning human bodies on industrial or proposed industrial sites. An important note here about all of the activists I interviewed and who participated in the think-aloud protocol is that all had identities outside of "environmental activist"; for example, all held employment outside of "environmental activism." Participants were wary of *simply* being labeled "an environmental activist," and also identified as family members, teachers, health care professionals, scientists, and scholars among other disciplines. Indeed, several mentioned during the interview or think-aloud protocol that the simplistic characterization of "environmental activists" presented a flattened view of complex civic discussions in which activists wished to engage. With the exception of three activists in New York and Pennsylvania each, the activists did not know each other (they might know of each other, but who were not aware of who might be participating in this study). While some had participated in environmental activist issues in the past, some participants found that this was the first time they negotiated local, state, and federal environmental risk participatory mechanisms. All did so because they perceived that they or their families were negatively impacted or stood to be negatively impacted, in some way, by the expansion of unconventional fossil fuel extraction and infrastructure.

In chapters 1 and 2, where I explore constraints felt by activists through rhetorical and CDA analysis, I continue to refer to participants as participants because many did not identify as activists until they felt stymied by institutional risk reporting. In chapters 3 and 4, I consciously make the switch to referring to participants as "activists" to highlight the ways in which public participants spoke, or continue to speak, about ways they might "oppose a dominant paradigm" (Cantrill, 1996, p. 168). Activists had voiced alarm at least once (but more often, several times), in a public space (either a concerned citizen's meeting[3] or a local or state institutional meeting) about working with institutional risk reporting tools that privilege the fossil fuel industry, in particular, the emerging technologies of hydraulic fracturing in the United States. These activists recognized that while participatory environmental risk assessments have been put into place in the United States, the very nature of underlying ideologies embedded in deliberative tools point to risk assessments that normalize dominant practices of fossil fuel energy extraction (as unconventional oil and gas production is a type of fossil fuel production). As such, understanding activists who propose alternatives to dominant discourses are particularly rich area of literacy study. Cantrill (1996) asserts that activist groups provide rich communicative scholarship potential because: "small grassroots alliances may exhibit the greatest rhetorical alienation exactly because they are often marginalized by more dominant cultural groupings" (p. 168).

In addition, as this study unfolded, it has been widely noted that human health grassroots activist efforts in the state of New York resulted in a statewide HVHF ban in December 2014 (note, HVHF infrastructure such as transport, storage, is still very much a contested issue in New York State); thus, some of my questions to New York participants were focused on their literate activities in getting the ban enacted (such bans do not extend to Pennsylvania or Ohio).

As this is a comparative study of participant literacies across three states, I chose not to include details of individual demographic information for each participant in this study for several reasons:

1. I wanted, and was bound to by the terms of my IRB, to protect the identity of participants who might have been arrested or who might have agreed to an anonymous interview and think-aloud protocol as an activist for the purposes of my study, but who might not want to identify as an activist in a more public setting.
2. As my analysis deepened the focus of my study, patterns about the ways in which participants were interacting with different institutional literacy processes or alternative processes made individual participant analysis less relevant to the goals of this study.

I was interested in the literate practices of activists who seek to expose the risks of fossil fuel technologies and literate practices that highlight deliberations allowing for alternatives to fossil fuels. For example, activists reported patterns of dissatisfaction in the way in which renewable energy discursive frames and sources are discouraged, implicitly or explicitly, in institutional environmental risk communication. I worked with several activist participants from each state who have shared literate artifacts[4] at public meetings or in a public setting (activist websites).

Activist artifacts included tools such as citizen action plans that outlined steps to discourage or interrupt local fossil fuel infrastructure by sharing model local ordinances, sharing emerging academic research, sharing local reports, and encouraging air, water, and human health baseline studies. Alternatively, citizen groups also shared steps for implementing local renewable energy infrastructure initiatives. These activists have worked with both institutional and alternative environmental risk analysis spaces. All activists participated in an interview and a think-aloud-protocol (TAP), and all shared risk information in a public setting as part of a community group concerned about environmental issues related to HVHF. In these meetings, the activists may have positioned themselves as spokespersons for a community group or as individuals informing communities about risk, depending on the public meeting. Some meetings had an agenda in which local community representatives presented, while other meetings allowed for questions or comments from individuals. In either scenario, participants shared personal anecdotes, scientific research, and strategies for community reporting models that are not included in institutional regulatory environmental agencies.

Specifically, data collection methods included the following:

(a) Interview: I conducted interviews before each think-aloud protocol to establish demographic and background knowledge and to learn about participants' practices engaging with institutionally sponsored risk reporting sites and procedures (local, state, and federal) and alternative risks reporting (how participants make knowledge about risk outside of institutionally sponsored risk reporting sites and procedures through contextualized, local knowledges). Interviews were "constructivist" in that the interviewer and interviewee co-constructed the direction of the conversation. Interviews included questions about how participants might navigate local, state, and federal risk reporting sites. Other questions detailed participants' literate practices as they navigating risk reporting sites that are not sponsored by local, state, and federal regulatory sites. (see appendix A)

(b) Think-aloud-protocols: I conducted two think-aloud protocols for each participant while participants navigated local, state, and federal risk

> reporting sites and non-institutional sites that discuss environmental risks (handouts, blogs, Facebook posts, citizen science documents, etc). I captured these navigations as screencast think-aloud recordings using Screen-Cast-O-Matic technologies (I recorded only the screens participants navigated, not the participants themselves). I conducted some think-aloud protocols in the homes of participants to observe participants' situated uses of literate practices. At other times, I conducted think-aloud protocols in a library or coffee shop at the participants' request (see appendix B).

Participants were free during the TAP or the interview to share any other public participatory mechanism from past experiences (whether it be online or in paper form) they might want to discuss. Finally, I often followed up interviews and TAPs by researching additional sources that might inform environmental policy deliberation mentioned by participants. For example, in each state, participants might mention advocacy groups, policy procedures, or historical precedents that I might research to understand participant interview or TAP responses more clearly (see appendix C).

During my observations, patterns of deliberation, often tied to difficulties in ways in which environmental risk information is shared (or not), began to emerge as participants reported, through the interview and TAP, issues of access *to* or *within* regulatory risk reporting tools. For example, concerned citizens in Ohio voiced frustration at the inability to contact a state regulatory reporting institution (such as the Ohio Department of Natural Resources, ODNR) to make a risk report about concerns of local HVHF injection wells, part of the HVHF process in which brine waste from HVHF is injected into underground wells. This led several in my study to identify themselves not only as concerned citizens but as "activists." Ohio activists used literate practices to navigate through the ODNR site; and, at times, citizen science participation in creating knowledge by contributing to emerging risk studies as related to injection wells (air, water and human health); activists navigated through state and local zoning laws and policies, through federal environmental laws and policies, and through renewable energy technologies and policies. Activists reported that these literate practices were often conducted in private, then shared in public forums, such as town hall meetings. Similarly, New York activists voiced concern about widespread infrastructure issues of expanded HVHF in the United States (gas lines, compressor stations, gas storage) that exist even if local HVHF production is banned. Literate practices were similar to those stated in Ohio, but the focus on risks to human health issues were noteworthy, as this public health frame (a critical discourse analysis consideration in terms of ideological "frames" in language), largely put forth by grassroots activists (rhetorical issue of authority, invention, and order), eventually led to a ban of the practice of hydraulic fracturing in New York.

CRITICAL LITERACIES AND ENVIRONMENTAL RISK ASSESSMENT

To be clear, this study looks at only a small part of environmental risk reporting within larger studies of communication; however, it does attend to the socially situated nature of this risk reporting. Past studies of environmental risk communication might include "psychometric methodologies" which explore how participants might use a particular tool without critical consideration of the tool in question. My study, which combines rhetorical analyses of contexts in which literate tools might be used, and critical discourse analysis of language found within literate tools themselves, looks closely and critically at the tools participants are being asked to use. This combination of rhetorical and critical discourse analysis is unique to my study and informs ways in which citizens might engage in risk meaning making to help to more clearly understand, as Grabill and Simmons point out, ways in which risk reporting tools might restrict citizens' roles in risk reporting by referring to critiques of a "decide-announce-defend" policy. (1998, p. 419). Simmons and Grabill argue that such policy excludes true public participation because "decision making (risk assessment) happens behind closed doors with risk communicators then charged with defending the decisions to a sometimes hostile public . . . soliciting public comment happens only after the real decisions have been made" (1998, p. 419).

Communication studies have typically resulted in technocratic and linear models that separate risk assessment and risk communication. This model results in the public being a "consumer" of information "rather than fostering an exchange and collaborative generation of knowledge that contributes to public policy" (Grabill and Simmons, 1998, p. 424). In response, I center this study on understanding the limitations of the public comment process in environmental risk deliberation.

My methodology, then, led me to consider analytical tools that can critique communication models that do not acknowledge the notion that risk is socially constructed. In addition, I sought tools that investigate patterns found within socially constructed models of environmental risk communication. My collection of user experiences with participatory mechanisms is underscored by an understanding of literacies embedded within the socially situated participatory process. Here, it is important to understand expanded notions of "usability." I again turn to Grabill and Simmons, who detail wider notions of usability than prescribed ways users might engage in literacies:

"we are looking toward a wider range of research practices—a range of contextual interviewing and observation practices in particular—that necessitate researchers work with audiences in the construction of knowledge (e.g., risk)." (1998, p. 431–432).

Grabill and Simmons also investigate ways "users" might move beyond texts that mediate particular orientations between humans and nature, and ways in which those who navigate these texts and spaces might participate within them: "users in all contexts are potential participants in decision-making about technologies—from computer interfaces and documentation to waste incinerators and construction projects. We feel they should be actual participants" (1998, p. 432). This notion of "usability" also allows me to explore an important pattern I found in my observations—that of issues of emerging or invented literacies used by activists that better suit a local, situated experience. I wanted to understand, more fully, how "users" might be "decision-makers." It is important to note that these literacies do not preclude literacies of technology or "science." Indeed, the activists may be scientists themselves who feel that institutional reporting does not represent specific scientific concerns.

When working with participants, I was guided by participants' navigations of environmental risk participatory mechanisms through interviews and TAPs to look specifically at local and state (and, at times, federal) representations of potential or existing environmental risk about energy production. I began to see patterns in participant interactions with institutional risk reporting and representational mechanisms in terms of participant reports of lack of or stymied participation. As I gathered my data, I took into account that much "public deliberation" occurs within physical meetings, but, more frequently, within online networks, which I represent through the TAP data collection in this dissertation. While my dissertation data collection was conducted through private TAP and interview sessions where I gathered, participants also reported recollections of ways in which they gathered and shared information about environmental risks in physical meetings. As such, I might move from various "streams" of language—from spoken and written representations of risk (Geisler, 2003). My focus for this study explored both institutionally sponsored risk reporting mechanisms as navigated by activists and alternatives created by activists to represent what they felt institutions were not representing.

METHODOLOGY AND METHODS

Concerned about environmental justice and precautionary policies, I ground my work in both critical action research and feminist research methods.

According to Blythe, Grabill, and Riley (2008), "action research is contextual, local, and requires intervention, not simply description" (p. 273). I attempt to avoid what Blythe, Grabill, and Porter caution researchers against: "using others for their own ends, such as publication" (p. 274). As such, I approached this research to more fully understand participant concerns versus my own preconceived notions of what their concerns might be.

My interest in social justice—particularly notions of environmental justice—underscores my orientation. My research methods are informed by scholarship surrounding "precautionary" risk reporting perspectives and practices, which could add significantly to the way in which stakeholders might contribute to environmental risk analysis (Whiteside, 2006). As detailed in the literature review, my study also explores frameworks of environmental justice that explore discursive possibilities, attending to expanded notions of citizen risk reporting in space and time (Holifield, Porter, and Walker, 2010; Walker, 2010; Nixon, 2011). Concepts like environmental justice challenge normate views of the environment and the relationships humans have with environmental spaces. Environmental justice frameworks seek expanded ideas about how places are labeled and how those living in geographically stigmatized spaces, as defined by dominant discourses, might find agency in redefining place and, by extension, personal identity. My concerns with environmental justice and precautionary risk reporting help to explain why I choose, for example, CDA as an analytical tool in addition to rhetorical analysis.

The notion of agency in defining a space, and potential risks in that space, is central to my study and informs my methodological choices within a feminist framework. Patricia Sullivan's (2012) discussion of the "reinterpretation" of composition scholarship involves a "metarhetorical" stance that allows me to explore a feminist critique of "methodological assumptions" within composition (p. 127). I extend such a critique to the literacies that public participants must navigate when attempting to voice an environmental concern. As noted in the literature review in chapter 1, particularly in the scholarship surrounding feminism, science, and sustainability, notions of "authority" to represent environmental risk show a wider scope of traditional notions of authority about the way in which knowledge is created and shared (Haraway, 1996; Harding, 1996; Warren, 2000; Sauer, 2003). However, while new ways of considering inclusivity might be theorized in the academy, I am led to question and learn about inclusivity occurring at the community level as public participants grapple with issues like hydraulic fracturing in their communities—at times, in their very backyards. As a member of a community impacted by the hydraulic fracturing industry myself, I have found identification with those that I study in terms of constraints of risk reporting in my own material environment, and I bring this viewpoint into my research design.

In reflecting upon my own experiences (and frustrations) in attempting to represent environmental risk in the state of Ohio, I think of Royster and Kirsch's (2012) notion of strategic contemplation where I might explore

> a space where we can see and hold contradictions without rushing to immediate closure, to neat resolutions, or to cozy hierarchies and binaries. The intent of such strategic contemplation is to render meaningfully, respectfully, honorably the words and works of those whom we study. (p. 21–22)

In my quest for such a reflective space in my own research, I draw from Grabill's (2012) articulations of community-based research, where researchers "draw on the practice of working with people to answer questions and solve problems, as opposed to researching 'on' people and their problem" (p. 212). During the interviews and think-aloud protocols in my study, where participants and I engaged in discussions about how they were navigating paper or technical documents, I take pointers from Selfe and Hawisher (2012) to contextualize the participants' literacy experiences by asking participants for "elaboration, encouraging them to reflect on stories they tell, and, occasionally, telling stories of (our) own when we find points in common" (p. 42). It is crucial for me to acknowledge the "contextual" and "situated" spaces where interventions are being composed, particularly in terms of online spaces where participants would gather or share information that was later shared in oral form in public meetings.

NOTES

1. Michael Halliday (1978) discusses semiotic or symbol systems that create linguistic meanings which are embedded in social processes, values, and actions. I define linguistic constructions in this study as patterns of linguistic symbols embedded in culture. These linguistic constructions might enable or limit the "meaning making potential" in knowledge making associated with environmental risks.
2. Literate artifacts used in this book relies on Witte's (2005) notion of mediating artifacts. A literate artifact can be considered to be reading or writing tools or technologies (networks of tools) that act as a medium to communicate (perform) within a certain social activity (activities are constantly in flux and interact with various other activity systems). Literate artifacts are socially situated.
3. Some activists attended concerned citizens meetings, but did not want neighbors or relatives to know they had attended these meetings. Others were quite public about their anti-fracking involvement.
4. Literate artifacts used in my study relies on Witte's (2005) notion of mediating artifacts. A literate artifact can be considered to be reading or writing tools or technologies (networks of tools) that act as a medium to communicate (perform) within a certain social activity (activities are constantly in flux and interact with various other activity systems). Literate artifacts are socially situated.

Chapter 1

Conflict

Stories of Language, Identity, Place, and Environmental Risk Practice

In this chapter, I examine patterns of deliberation, public participant agency, and place. More just technical communication is not a matter of simply changing technical language on a website. As my analysis shows, there is a disparity in uneven access to how different stakeholders deliberate about environmental concerns in different geographical areas and what agency they have to protect environmental and human health. For example, my past research details how the lack of public participation in the HVHF industry has had disproportionate impacts on residents who live near HVHF industry sites, such as areas of Appalachia, including Southwestern PA. These places have histories of extractive economies and poverty and, currently, lack the agency to speak about environmental justice and intersectional concerns (George, 2019b).

The disparities of HVHF health concerns are highlighted when considering that an adjacent state, New York, placed a ban on HVHF drilling, largely informed by a public health argument based on recommendations from the New York Department of Health. How could definitions of HVHF risk and attendant policy vary across state lines and across two state health departments (George, 2019b)?

While New York banned the practice of drilling on the basis of a human health argument, in Pennsylvania, a state gag order, Act 13, enacted in 2012, initially did not allow for the disclosure of HVHF chemicals to doctors in cases of suspected exposure. While several provisions of Act 13 were struck down by a 2016 Pennsylvania Supreme Court ruling, years of positioning economic interests above unknown human health effects informed a green light for industry versus precautionary practice (Philips, 2016). The result is an instance of "slow violence" (Nixon, 2013) that manifest in human bodies—often in poor rural areas with a history of past exploitive carbon extraction practices. These places and bodies serve as collateral damage to the advancement of the HVHF industry. While the current governor of Pennsylvania, Tom Wolfe, has recently called for public health studies related to HVHF, this is only after an outcry based on an increase of a variety of other widely publicized health studies that suggest HVHF causes a litany of health issues: childhood cancers, low infant birth rates, and so on. In the meanwhile, several chemicals used in HVHF activity are still protected from public knowledge, and powerful interests maintain the status quo of drilling. "The Marcellus Shale Coalition, a gas industry group, maintains there is no credible link between fracking and childhood cancers" (Tanenbaum, 2019).

HISTORICAL CONCEPT OF "ENVIRONMENTAL IDENTITIES" IN EACH STATE

In this study, I posit that perceptions and representations of risk are socially constructed, so it is important to have some understanding of the similarities and differences in the histories of environmental risk regulation and policy in the states of the participants that I chose to study: New York, Pennsylvania, and Ohio. My central question, *How do public participants engage in and take part in risk communication and deliberation about environmental risk and energy policy*, rests upon the notion that varied ideologies create particular policies and practices in regards to environmental risk. It is not simply by studying the geography and geology of a particular space itself, but ideas about how humans (or other organisms) might interact within an environment that indicate particular policies and practices. These three states are all share an industrial past; portions of each of these states identify as the "Rust Belt" and have experienced a decline from heavy industrial manufacturing, though those declines vary within each state. The three states also touch upon a vast natural entity: Lake Erie, which historically enabled much industrial activity. Buffalo, NY, Erie, PA, and Cleveland, OH are within a 200-mile radius and share the Lake Erie shoreline. Additionally, each state continues to provide a significant contribution to agriculture production.

However, a historical overview of environmental movements in each state shows past patterns of resource use and conservation has, to some degree, impacted where and how HVHF occurs in each state and how public participants from each state can navigate literacies related to HVHF (Finewood and Stroup, 2012). Stibbe (2015) argues that "identity" in the social and personal senses of the word create models for humans that orient them toward particular ideologies about their relationship with concepts like "nature" or the "environment." These orientations are manifested through behavior and are recursively reinforced through texts and social systems (Stibbe, 2015, p.

107–108). Particular attitudes about humans and their relationship to their environment were revealed more clearly through rhetorical and discourse investigations as participants worked through literate practices. I contend these attitudes are deeply tied to an understanding of regional identities and the history of that identity that link to values and action about HVHF. During my pilot investigations, I found that it was important to situate the study around the histories of state natural and environmental movements as related to policy and practice in each state, as these attitudes reflected various positions about energy development and HVHF. Note, while there is considerable Native American and geological history that should be and are acknowledged in geological, environmental history, and postcolonial studies, that investigation is outside the scope of this study. The general storyline of Western perceptions and constructs of "nature" or "the environment" in American literature and art moves through early colonial writing that often represents the taming of a wilderness, to the Romantic period, where "nature" is often seen as "the sublime," to the more recent modern-day environmental movement (Dryzek, 2005). Against this rather simplistic and normative understanding of American relation to nature, each state in my study offers a different frame depending upon varying broad historical patterns that show deep differences in relations between humans and the natural environment through time and space.

NEW YORK—ENVIRONMENT AS WILDERNESS

It was clear to me, going into this research, that stakeholders could find purchase and agency with a powerful cultural framing of nature as found in the well-documented history of the Adirondack region. Understanding environmental policy history in New York shows the emergence of a particular discursive approach to "nature." It is interesting to note that the Adirondacks comprise a large geographic area of the state devoted to "wilderness."

The roots of the American Romantic movement, in which nature is seen as something of a "sublime" force, are well documented in New York's historic collected writing and visual art. This is particularly clear in highly influential romantic odes to the Adirondacks and the Catskills, where nature is often depicted as "pristine," with an inherent value in aesthetics versus only a resource value (Edmonson, 2001, p. 9). Most notable are the ways in which influential American writers and artists from New York, or who centered work about New York, established an identity, through writing and art, beyond that of the European "civility"—to an American concept of "wilderness" (p. 9).[1] Additionally, a variety of pragmatic social forces in the nineteenth century merged to create notions of "nature" that resulted in a "forever wild" designation of portions of

New York's forests as early as 1894 (Edmonson, 2001). Successive decades found expanded parks and public lands, particularly in western New York, initially fueled by sporting groups and wealthy tourists, where wilderness was largely discursively framed as enabling recreational activity and where nature might be enjoyed for aesthetic value (Dryzek, 2005). The ways in which influential New York literary and artistic works led to American notions of aesthetic and recreational "wilderness" are important to note because these designations led to designations of "wild" space policies that reverberated far beyond the borders of New York State. According to Edmonson, Olmstead's radical notion (at the time) of Central Park (1858) as a place of aesthetic respite expanded to his influence in advocating for Yosemite as a state park in 1863 (2001, p. 9). New York also led the nation in establishing forestry schools in the state public universities. Here, the conservation focus shifted from aesthetics, viewing wilderness as a resource that must be managed (Dryzek, 2005), but by the 1960s and 1970s, the intrinsic value of nature had asserted itself firmly in the New York region, according to Edmonson (2001).

But what is most compelling for this study is the way in which New York State's environmental positioning and policies have had a long history of balancing relationships between human health, economic health, and natural systems, particularly between large metropolises and the designation of natural areas (Stradling, 2010; Davies, 2013). Edmonson (2001) traces several urban epidemic outbreaks in rapidly growing industrial cities in New York in the late 1800s. The rise of relatively cheap railway transportation from New York City to rural areas like Saranac Lake in the Adirondacks led to tuberculosis cures and the establishment of sanitariums, which created particularly powerful ideas between the importance of "pristine nature" and "public health." "The opinions of physicians like Trudeau and Chapin helped solidify the public's belief that human health was enhanced by clean water and fresh air, and that mental health was aided by access to rural tranquility" (Edmondson, 2001, p. 12). Similarly, Edmonson notes other important developments in the late 1800s in New York State's relationship with nature and forest conservation via State Forest Preserve and "wild" designations, which were based on an argument for both drinking water and industry for canals: "The water argument was particularly compelling as it was predicated upon on the symbiotic relationship between natural areas with finite resources, economic capital and expanding populations in New York cities" (2001, p. 12). The way in which New York's environmental legislation took form is crucial to this study as it resulted in groups coalescing to define particular environmental notions of space within state policy:

> It was one of the first times that state law-makers were persuaded by the opinions of naturalists and scientists. Most significant, it established the precedent

> that protecting water, soil, and timber resources were public goals that could override private property rights. (p. 12)

New York State continues this advocacy for preservation and conservation of nature:

> Throughout the state of New York, law groups, activist groups, foundations, and smaller donors have developed well-organized systems that can act rapidly to protect land and pass environmental legislation around the globe. To a great extent, the headquarters of this cartel is in New York City. (Edmonson, 2001, p. 40)

According to Edmonson, citizen's environmental groups have had a documented practice of pushing back against expert scientists employed by industry.

This is not to say that New York was and is immune from environmental risk. Of interest to the areas I chose to study in this dissertation is the notion of socially constructed borders and social practices within borders. Protection of the Adirondack forests from the phenomena of acid rain led New York scientists in the 1970s to conclude that risks emerged from other places. Acid rain "came from the industrial Midwest, especially the tall-stacked coal-fired plants of the Ohio Valley" (Stradling, 2010, p. 220). New York scientists and politicians were among the first to advocate for a series of federal laws and amendments aimed at reducing sulfur and nitrogen emissions in the next two decades, resulting in the 1990 creation of the Acid Rain Program under the Clean Air Act to manage acid rain (Stradling, 2010, p. 220–222). In the late 1970s, Love Canal, an environmental and public health disaster that was the result of improper storage of toxic waste from the declining industries, namely Hooker Chemical Company (Edmondson, 2001, p. 48). The disaster made the efforts of Lois Gibbs, a local stakeholder who became a chemical risk expert, a national name (Stradling, 2010). Love Canal's cleanup led to highly influential hazardous waste regulations on a state and federal level, including the Comprehensive Environmental Response, Compensation, and Liability Act (CERCLA) or Superfund Act, which provides funds for the cleaning up of toxic waste sites, and EPA laws which required that industry be partially responsible for unknown risks (Stradling, 2010; Edmonson, 2001). Given the nature of environmental advocacy and agency in New York State, it was not surprising that, during my data collection, New York passed a ban against HFHV drilling activity.

PENNSYLVANIA—ENVIRONMENT AS RESOURCE AND RECREATION

It is noteworthy that, unlike NY, where there are several sources of environmental history, there is simply less established research about the environmental movements in the state of PA. In 1999, Joel Tarr made an observation about the lack of documentation of Pennsylvania's environmental history: "there has been relatively little written on the topic . . . until recently, the Commonwealth's colleges and universities did not have environmental historians on their faculty" (p. 445).

There are several well-known environmentalists with ties to Pennsylvania, but many of them found notoriety in leaving Pennsylvania. For example, Philadelphians John and William Bertram's botanical work stems from extensive travel through the United States and beyond. Rachel Carson was born in and attended college in Pittsburgh, but studied and wrote about coastal waterways and had long settled in Maryland before publishing the highly influential *Silent Spring* (this text was published in Boston). This lack of general recognition of environmental historical research in Pennsylvania underscores the ways in which Pennsylvania's natural identity is often seen, rather narrowly, in terms of carbon extraction. According to Hardy, highly influential energy extraction is inextricable from the history of both the eastern and western portions of this state:

> Nowhere in the United States can the history of energy regimes—the sources of energy that fuel our lives and economies—be better told than in Pennsylvania. The Commonwealth was home to more than 95 percent of the anthracite coal in the Western Hemisphere and vast deposits of bituminous coal, the birthplace of the world oil industry (Titusville, 1859), the first successful three-wire electric lighting system in the United States (Sunbury in 1883), the world's first large-scale nuclear power plant (Shippingport, 1957), and the nation's worst nuclear accident. (Three Mile Island, 1979) (2012, p. 477)

Environmental history scholars discuss the historical significance of pollution as a result of resource extraction in Pennsylvania by revealing the historical patterns that led to industrial growth from Pennsylvania's natural resources that allowed for "unprecedented wealth" which was largely moved "into the hands of an industrial elite" (Hardy, 2012, p. 481). However, this wealth, according to Hardy, was in stark contrast to struggling coal, mill, and lumber towns that are still recovering from the end of extractive economies (2012, p. 481). Similarly, Black and Ladson discuss the historical impacts of energy extraction history in Pennsylvania by focusing on the changes in social patterns that enabled carbon extraction: "the mountains of Pennsylvania were now viewed as a great vault for carbon" (2012, p. 378). This carbon extraction was ubiquitous in the state, as were the accompanying social inequities that continue to be a part of this carbon extraction where the environment was seen largely as a resource, "the transformation of the Appalachians in Pennsylvania into the nation's greatest energy landscape also came with significant residual costs attached" (2012, p. 378).

The lack of general recognition of environmental historical research in Pennsylvania underscores the ways in which Pennsylvania's natural identity is often seen, rather narrowly, in terms of carbon extraction.

Much of the "story" of the documented historical Pennsylvania environment relies on carbon extraction and the state and federal policies that exist today in response to the pollution from that extraction. Industrial pollution was simply part of the makeup of Pennsylvania cities as extractive industries progressed, but concerted policies to control it were not often put into place until after large-scale public health damage (Hardy, 2012; Black and Ladson, 2012).

Susan Comfort's (2017) work with HVHF activists in southwest PA coal country finds strong identity and discursive ties to the carbon extraction past and the ways in which systems to perpetuate carbon extraction might hold purchase, despite intersectional risks of past extraction.[2]

Much of the "story" of the documented historical Pennsylvania environment relies on carbon extraction and the state and federal policies that exist today in response to the pollution from that extraction. Industrial pollution was simply part of the makeup of Pennsylvania cities as extractive industries progressed, but concerted policies to control it were not often put into place until after large-scale public health damage. According to Hardy, the Donora Smog, which occurred on October 29, 1948, had devastating effects for a small town of Donora to the south of Pittsburgh:

> It was the smog inversion that blanketed the nearby milltown of Donora in 1948, sickening seven thousand and killing twenty, which shocked Americans and impelled Congress to pass the first national legislation to limit air pollution: the Clean Air Act of 1955. (2012, p. 484)

Similarly, Pennsylvania continues to grapple with issues related to abandoned mine land throughout the state, including water quality issues, acid mine drainage, and the struggle for larger economic redevelopment. The federal Surface Mine Control and Reclamation Act (SMCRA) was passed in 1977 to address past mine abandonment by establishing reclamation funds by taxing the coal industry and to implement regulations for future mining. However, the implementation of such laws is often ambiguous, and thousands of acres of abandoned mine land in Pennsylvania remain. The marginalization of Pennsylvania's landscape have given rise to some local advocacy groups like the Pennsylvania Center for Coalfield Justice to help public participants to navigate both coal and HVHF regulatory policies and engage in networks between state and local economic initiatives to reimagine abandoned mine lands (Abandoned Mine Reclamation Clearinghouse; "What We Do"; "Center for Coalfield Justice"). The marginalization of Pennsylvania's landscape have given rise to some local advocacy groups like the Southwest Pennsylvania Environmental Health Project, which defines itself as follows: "The Environmental Health Project (EHP) is a nonprofit public health organization that assists and supports residents of Southwestern Pennsylvania and beyond who believe their health has been, or could be, impacted by unconventional oil and gas development" (UOGD, or fracking) (Southwest Environmental Health Project, 2021, About EHP) who seek a concerted public health response in spite of "the lack of objective, reliable data on the health effects of UOGD activities raises many questions about the origins of residents' health problems and the scope of public health risks in communities" (Southwest Environmental Health Project, 2021 About EHP). Another important note is that due to the Halliburton Loophole in the Energy Act of 2005, these SMCRA regulations do not apply to HVHF drilling or storage operations, sparking a concern by many stakeholders about intersectional or layered risks of multiple industries through space and time. In an ironic twist, there are many places in Pennsylvania where HVHF operations exist beside or within acid mine drainage restoration sites. George (2017a, 2017b) argues that language embedded in environmental narratives of technocratic "corrections" to past industrial activity, particularly in marginalized landscapes, makes assumptions that layered "risks" can be managed.

However, amid a narrative of extraction, scholars do argue that there have been strong conservation forces in Pennsylvania in vast forest acquisition through the efforts of well-known conservationists like Joseph Rothrock in the late 1800s and Gifford Pinchot, who led the new U.S. Forest service project in 1904. By 2000, Pennsylvania state forestland reached four million acres, which is a substantial acreage compared to adjacent states (Hardy, 2012, p. 487). However, those acres were not necessarily framed as either space for recreation or pristine nature. Cutcliffe notes that Pinchot's rhetoric for conservation is based on the notion of how forests might serve humans. "Pinchot was largely responsible for developing a 'wise use,' utilitarian approach to managing natural resources that set aside increasing amounts of national forest land for potential productive future use" (2012, p. 602). While New York certainly shares this utilitarian approach as well, the early framing of New York's "wilderness" areas offer different orientations to "nature."

While Pennsylvania's environmental identity is deeply entwined with its history of energy extraction, the current drilling activity in the northeast and southwest portions of the state is heavily drilled as compared to the available HVHF shale play. Here, we consider concepts from chapter 1, such as the geographic distribution of risk—partly dictated by the geography of the state (energy-producing shale largely follows the extraction). But partly due to the way in which the possible recoverable shale gas is in the Chesapeake Bay Watershed, which has largely been protected by the Chesapeake Bay Foundation (CBF), supported by federal, not state, EPA guidelines and laws:

> U.S. Environmental Protection Agency (EPA) signed the first of many inter-jurisdictional agreements with Maryland, Virginia, Pennsylvania, and the District of Columbia. The partners recognized the need for cooperative action if the Chesapeake Bay were ever to be removed from EPA's "dirty waters" list. (Chesapeake Bay Foundation, "Pollution Limits by State")

Specifically, the agency of the CBF, a multistate initiative, has clear statements about the watersheds of Central and Southeast PA that flow into water that is bordered by other states—and how this impacts the practice of HVHF drilling in Pennsylvania. Whereas the CBF takes pains not to disparage the HVHF industry as a whole, the information about HVHF found on the CBF site suggests a more precautionary approach and point specifically to precaution in Pennsylvania in terms of the HVHF industry:

> Instead, we have embraced the precautionary principle. Our over-arching goal is to ensure that future energy development in the Chesapeake Bay region takes place in as safe and environmentally responsible a manner as possible. We have joined others in calling for a federal study of cumulative impacts of Marcellus shale development in the region and active participation in state policy initiatives. (Chesapeake Bay Foundation, "Natural Gas")

Pennsylvania is an important state to review in terms of this study in that public participants have varied agency to deliberate about HVHF in certain parts of the state. Because of relationships and agreements about "nature" in terms of a multistate effort to restore the health of the Chesapeake Bay, Pennsylvania participants in the Chesapeake Bay watershed might deliberate within particular environmental frames that discourage HVHF activity.

OHIO—ENVIRONMENT AS RESOURCE

Of the three states I chose for this study, Ohio has the least amount of environmental history scholarship available; the existing scholarship tends to focus on geological features as well as some notable state naturalists (Lafferty, 1979). Despite the lack of a more robust environmental history scholarship archive, Ohio certainly offers a history of natural "spaces" in terms of parks and wildlife areas. Many of these spaces have been consciously created as a respite from industry, as modeled by other cities. For example, the "Emerald Necklace" Metropolitan Park System in Cleveland "may have been influenced by Boston's Emerald Necklace" (Sisson, 2012). Boston's system of city parks was designed by Olmstead, the influential parks visionary mentioned in the New York section of this chapter. The Cuyahoga Valley National Park is another notable conservation area in the state of Ohio.

However, Ohio's geological features factor into other ways in which agriculture has impacted the landscape. Unlike New York or Pennsylvania, the "relatively flat" geography in the north of the state is more suited to farmland (Easterling and Karl, 2001). As a result, Ohio, which was once largely covered in forest, has fewer wooded areas per acre than either Pennsylvania or New York. In fact, Ohio differs significantly in forest cover and its history of forest conservation. All three states were once were predominately covered with forests. All three states were heavily timbered over time, but whereas Pennsylvania and New York states currently have forest cover at or slightly above 50 percent, Ohio, which once stood as the western "wild" frontier of the nation, currently has a forest cover that rests at slightly above 30 percent (USDA Forest Service). Most of these Ohio forests exist in the southern part of the state, which currently includes initiatives to reforest previously strip-mined lands ("History of Ohio's State Forests").

Along with agriculture, Ohio, like Pennsylvania, has seen significant energy extraction in the east and south in the form of coal, gas, and oil. But it was the rise of industry and manufacturing throughout most of the twentieth century that defined many Ohio cities. Equally important are the ways in which declines in manufacturing hit Ohio's identity particularly hard ("Early Industrialization"; "Business and Industry"). Ohio's relation with declining industry is often marked by the burning Cuyahoga River in 1969. To be clear, the Cuyahoga had burned several times before—and states such as Pennsylvania and Michigan also experienced "burning rivers" (Adler, 2004, p. 95). But the media attention given to the Cuyahoga in 1969 which sparked the creation of the modern water protections such as the Clean Water Act of 1970. The burning Cuyahoga River, along with several other events that were widely covered by media at the time, such as the wide reporting of the "death" of Lake Erie, which borders Ohio, gave rise, in part, to the development of the EPA (Stradling and Stradling, 2008; Davies, 2013). The notion of Ohio's troubled waters persists, particularly in media cycles. Despite some protections, as recently as 2014, Ohio's governor declared a state of emergency due to algal blooms from farming that resulted in toxins in the water in the Toledo region (Yeoman, 2014).

While there is some multistate and international (Canada) cooperation in Ohio with the Great Lakes Restoration Initiative, which was launched in 2010, there is no statement from the Great Lakes Restoration Initiative literature about how HVHF activity might complicate the mission of the Great Lakes Restoration Initiative ("Great Lakes"). As noted earlier in this chapter, industry in the "Midwest," including Ohio, was often seen as the genesis of acid rain that affected other states as a result of sulfur dioxide emissions from coal-fired plants. Policies to curb these emissions have largely come from the federal, not state level (Stradling, 2010).

More recently, Ohio has come to the forefront in yet another environmental disaster. The Norfolk Southern train derailment in East Palestine, Ohio, on February 3, 2023, released a toxic mix of chemicals including vinyl chloride and hydrogen chloride into the air and water of nearby communities. Some called it the worst human-caused environmental disaster since Chernobyl.

The City of East Palestine issued a press release on February 5, declaring that "Our drinking water is safe for residents," and Mike DeWine, governor of Ohio, declared that residents could safely return to their homes on February 8, just five days after the derailment. However, mitigation of the chemical spill site has involved physically removing truckloads of dirt, homes have undergone re-entry screenings and well testing by the EPA to assure residents of their safety, and the state opened up a permanent health clinic to support the future health needs of residents following the chemical exposure. These actions contradict the purported safety of the town and its residents.

Current State Identities—Energy

These state environmental histories help to inform current policy positions about energy production in each state; this history also helps to explain participatory mechanisms in place by varied state institutions. While the three states have and continue to account for significant energy production and consumption rates in the United States, investigating *how* the three states produce and consume energy is an important consideration for this study in terms of the ways in which participants' literate practices respond to these patterns in the production and consumption of HVHF and environmental risk. The Energy Information Administration, or EIA, in 2014 reported that technological advancements in hydraulic fracturing allows for significant *potential* gas production in each of these states; however, legislation that bans HVHF drilling in NY has dropped possible projections in NY. As of 2021, the EIA projects overall shale gas production to continue in Ohio and Pennsylvania into the future. Pennsylvania is currently one of the top producers in the United States (2021). The results of such production have, according to the EIA (2014), resulted in the United States at that time emerging as the largest petroleum and natural gas producer in the world in 2014, which has been supplanted only by China by 2021. As noted in New York's ban, questions and research about environmental risks of HVHF arise, practices related to hydraulic fractured energy production might be interrupted (such as the HVHF ban in New York); "inevitable" futures that include hydraulic fracturing production projections are called into question. My pilot data revealed that citizens might attempt to counter this inevitability by presenting local risk (air or water quality) and global risk (global climate change) through institutional environmental risk reporting mechanisms, or by finding alternative literacies to represent risk. The question of citizens' agency in any attempt to present environmental risk largely depends upon a variety of social factors for a given citizen in a particular state or even a particular location within a state. My study focuses on how citizen literacies and deliberation in each of these states shape risk assessments that influence environmental policies related to energy deliberation. Because of the Energy Act of 2005, HVHF is largely exempt from federal regulation. According to Brady, "The bulk of the regulatory responsibility is given to the several states, and these regulations vary widely in their complexity and level of protection of human health and the environment" (2011, p. 18).

As regulation of HVHF falls to states, each state's policies show different possibilities for citizen engagement in defining and reporting potential energy risks that stem from hydraulic fracturing and energy production, so citizen engagement and use of literacy to attempt to define HVHF risks vary by each state (Brady, 2011; Kear, 2011; Kear and Forbis, 2015).

What happens when comparing policies that stakeholders and citizens in different states interact with? For example, Ohio's State Bill 310, passed in June of 2014 after widespread hydraulic fracturing infrastructure and production was implemented in the state, "freezes" a wide portion of alternative energy implementation. This is contrasted sharply with New York's ban on hydraulic fracturing in December of 2014. The comparison shows policies that shape varied energy ideologies that impact citizens who attempt to represent HVHF risk. Similarly, what emerges when comparing each state in terms of defining hazardous waste risk and policy? Varied definitions result in discrepancies in which some states are encouraged to accept hydraulic fracturing brine water injection wells, while other states' policies ban this practice and send the waste to neighboring states. As I explored these emerging inconsistencies across states in my pilot data, I also began to pursue research about the technical literacies participants must navigate in identifying and representing environmental risk. Research about community use of technical "civic commons" and technical documents used by citizens in participatory environmental discussions highlight various "ways" of presenting discourse about risk.

NOTES

1. Edmonson (2001) and Nash (1968) point to the following influential environmental writers and artists who either used New York as subject matter, worked in, or were from New York: Rene de Chateaubriand (1791–92); Charles Feno Hoffman (1836); Joel T. Headley (1849); James Fenimore Cooper (1823–1842 via various series); Thomas Cole (beginning in 1825), Hudson River School, with students Frederick Church and Arthur B. Durand; Ralph Waldo Emerson's poem: "The Adirondacks," 1858; John Burroughs, (beginning in 1871). Note, extensive postcolonial scholarship has pointed to a variety of visual artists and writers who have expanded notions of "nature" and "wilderness."

2. Comfort's scholarship reveals how communities who identify as "coal communities" frame the past (she outlines coal "heritage" days in several coal communities) and how this framing of past activity links to continued carbon extraction via HVHF activity in these locales. Her scholarship details how current HVHF operations often appeal to a nostalgic past, where coal extraction might be viewed in sentimental terms. Comfort suggests these "pasts" are largely fictional, as most communities were essentially colonized by larger industries at significant environmental and economic costs.

Chapter 2

Frames

Stories of Environmental Regulatory Bodies and Attempts to Deliberate about Risk

Both rhetorical and ecolinguistic scholarship are important in this study in terms of understanding the deliberative possibilities in which citizens might participate, most notably by exploring notions of authority or ethos in environmental public policy discussion. I am principally concerned about the ways in which various players with various persuasive goals frame notions of "science" and "risk." Studies in rhetoric also help to outline the pattern of policy formation about a given risk. The rhetorical notion of stasis is particularly helpful to trace risk formation as varied actors deliberate about whether phenomena are indeed risks, what the risks are, and what policies and practices might (or might not) emerge from these definitions.

DELIBERATION: PARTICIPATORY RISK MECHANISMS THROUGH ENVIRONMENTAL RISK ASSESSMENTS

Critical discourse analysis (CDA) reveals ideologies that are embedded in the language of environmental risk frames, particularly those legitimized in institutional environmental risk participatory mechanisms. These frames are found in specific texts, documents, and processes citizens use to participate in understanding and reporting environmental risks. As noted earlier in the chapter, concepts of risk are socially constructed through discursive frames, or shared ways of apprehending the world. CDA is particularly helpful in tracing ideological agency or legitimation of particularly powerful discursive frames.

Finally, as actors struggle to make meaning within institutionalized framing of risk, understanding the ways in which rhetorical "invention" emerges in risk representation is particularly important. Participants often "invent" using an expanded understanding of their authority and emerging digital technologies to participate in environmental risk deliberation, which I explore later in this book. This notion of participant authority is informed by emerging scholarship on situated literate practices of individuals, in this case stakeholders who seek to work within and sometimes beyond regulatory risk reporting tools sponsored by institutions.

Additionally, rhetorical studies are integral to my study because rhetorical analysis reveals important patterns of persuasion in a socially situated public sphere. In a call for rhetoric for "civic discourse in policy debates," Simmons (2007) encourages public space to be made available for complex and technical deliberation: "Technically complex public issues complicated the traditional notion of discourse because technical experts claim ownership of the technical issues and close off public debate even though these issues affect the public in very concrete ways" (p. 4). In my study, I am ultimately concerned with citizens' navigations through regulatory risk reporting tools. How do citizens read and write to negotiate these deliberative spaces? These are spaces where, ideally, actors can deliberate in an attempt to achieve consensus about environmental risks. I am interested in the authority by which institutional participatory mechanisms (public hearings, public surveys, etc.) and risk reporting tools (texts and procedures) emerge and are maintained within deliberative spaces. This public deliberative space must be addressed: who has the authority to speak in these spaces, and how are certain ideologies privileged in these spaces? Finding a deliberative space to examine issues of complex environmental risk is difficult, partly because of the struggle in determining who might have "true" authority or expertise to engage in these deliberations. Environmental risk scholars suggest risk representations are socially situated and socially contested (Beck, 1987; Lash, Szerszynski, and Wynne, 1996; Sauer, 2003). I apply this notion of socially constructed risk to HVHF environmental risk construction through a rhetorical approach: I interrogate *who* is making risk assessments that lead to policy. When environmental risk assessment[1] is linked to science (as it often is), an emerging body of work exploring rhetorics of science reveals nuances of authority, ethos, and the descriptive or prescriptive approaches to science and policy. Here, I note the historical divide in science between knowledge claims and policy. The way in which science claims are used by different actors to establish authority, particularly in environmental studies, makes "science" an important area of rhetorical investigation in understanding environmental risk assessment and policy. Whose "science" speaks for what particular environmental policy?

Rhetorical scholarship has attended to these issues of authority and deliberation by investigating, more clearly, values underlying science policy formation, but few rhetorical studies have investigated HVHF policy formation. As such, I ground my rhetorical analysis in what Edward Schiappa (1993) refers to as an "is/ought" construction to more clearly uncover authority in policy formation.[2] For example, Schiappa emphasizes the "is/ought" construction by discussing socially constructed definitional concerns that lead to the "ought" or the ways in which particular linguistic definitions might shape particular behaviors:

> The proponent seeks to change our linguistic behavior and thereby alter patterns of denotative conformity. Accordingly, the question arguers should be asking is not "What is X?" but rather "How ought we use the word X?" or "What should be described by the word X?" Normative questions of this sort cannot be answered acontextually; they virtually compel interlocutors to address the pragmatic needs of a given community of language-users located in a particular historical moment. Viewed rhetorically, proponents of new definitions seek to alter the behavior of a specific audience. (1998, p. 18)

Schiappa suggests that it is important to understand definitions of consequence (the *is*) that have been "empowered" through the ways in which social understandings of definitions emerge: "Such responses may be shaped through the application of various forms of power from logical or moral suasion, through bribery, to coercion" (Sederberg, 1984, p. 7) (1998, p. 20). With the interests in my study, I attend to Schiappa's question of the authority to determine what *is,* and what *ought* to be, a sociopolitical concern.

Schiappa uses an environmental example of "is" and "ought" construction by pointing to the designation of "wetlands" as a socially constructed and political definition. Schiappa reviews a historical shift in the way "wetlands" designations have become valued politically. Contested definitions of "wetlands" were codified to create a standard ecological definition of wetlands to serve policy and institutions[3] that increasingly saw value in these once marginalized lands (1998, p. 24–26). However, despite an ecological definition, Schiappa outlines continued contestation of wetland value and policy deliberation that led to competing questions among scientific experts and politicians about how wetlands might be designated and protected (1998, p. 32–36). Schiappa's discussion of ways in which complex systems like wetlands might be defined, contested, and protected by various actors are important to environmental language study because it underscores the ways in which socially constructed definitions informed by particular values of actors lead to specific policies and actions that result from policies.

In my study, I argue that it is in analyzing ways in which the *is* is defined by various actors in HVHF risk that leads to understanding the ways socially situated assumptions of values often appear in discussions of risk, and, by extension, the *ought*, of the HVHF policies informed by these definitions.

COMPETING SCIENCE CLAIMS AND HVHF DISCOURSE

But my participant data also reveals with the ways in which varied branches of expert science is often invoked in the attempt to legitimate HVHF activity, particularly in Pennsylvania and Ohio. When scientific stakeholders enter into technical discussions, which Lefsrud and Meyer (2012) refer to as "boundary work," they do so with varied interests that "contend for, legitimate, or challenge the cognitive authority of– and the credibility, prestige, power, and material resources that attend such a position [science]." (2012, p. 1480). This "boundary work" concept applies to notions of "agency capture" (Cox, 2006) or "weak" ecological modernization (Dryzek, 2005) in which industry places pressure on decision-makers (policy scientists) to influence regulatory decisions in favor of industry. Discourse scholars suggest that "science" that has been "captured," or "co-opted" by powerful ideologies cannot represent citizens' concerns at large. Added to this concern is the way in which such pro-industry science positioning does not recognize complex risk in terms of precaution: "The precautionary principle applies especially in situations of environmental risk where by the time unambiguous scientific evidence of a serious problem becomes available, the danger may have already have materialized and perhaps become irreversible" (Whiteside, 2006, p. viii). This notion of ideologies informing different definitions of risk highlights Frank Fischer's concerns about ideologies that underscore environmental policy:

> the production of knowledge about environmental problems and the subsequent policy responses are more a function of political and economic power than "objective science," and that leaving decisions up to "the experts" is simply a recipe for furthering the interests of corporate and state elites at the expense of both ordinary citizens and the environment. (2000, p. 263–264)

Another interpretation of "boundary work" is the ways in which varied science constructs, especially as related to the "environment," are often an amalgam of several branches of sciences. Such acknowledgment, though complex and nonlinear, offers alternative representations of environmental risks. Herndl and Cutlip (2013) discuss Kuhn's revolutionary work in exposing the limitations of absolutist objective "positivistic" truths. Fischer calls for social studies of science to adopt epistemological post-positivist approaches that "situates empirical inquiry in a broader interpretive framework" to complex social issues, such as environmental risk assessment (1998, p. 129). Similarly, Functowicz and Ravetz (1993) consider the way in which socially constructed notions of uncertainty complicates past "normal" positivist science philosophies. Of central importance to my study is their attention to the use of extended peer communities to address complex, costly, and potentially lethal uncertainties. This scholarship has informed more recent work in sustainability studies, which links knowledge-making across disciplines through "complex theories" which increase "validity" in addressing complicated issues (Wells, 2013). Sustainable science, in general, is concerned with the emergence of more complex notions of science and decision-making (McGreavy, Silka, and Hart, 2012).

In response to the emergence of sustainability studies, several researchers call for rhetorics to promote public deliberation in the interest of a "sustainable future." These rhetorics might acknowledge possible deliberative spaces among varied authorities and varied ideological frameworks that are central to my study, yet few offer empirical examples that showcase ways varied authorities might deliberate, a focus of my study. (Goggin, 2009; Buizer, Arts, and Kok, 2011; Scholz, 2011). Of course what, exactly, is to be "sustained" is debatable and is at times suspect, as Goggin (2009) acknowledges. However, "sustainable" deliberative constructs have shown new rhetorical approaches to policy-making in that both scientific inquiry and a wider participant base may both be used in the formation of making knowledge, a key investigative concern in my study. Similarly, Kuhn's work has informed the scholarship of feminist science scholars, such as those in Keller and Longino's (1996) edited collection, *Feminism and Science*, which have called for more situated studies of science and more complicated notions of "objectivity" and "reflexivity" in science (Haraway, 1996; Harding, 1996). Karen Warren's work (2000), *Ecofeminist Philosophy* explores conceptual intersections between feminism, science, and nature and argues for deliberative spaces about environmental risks that more clearly challenge oppressive deliberative practices to create more just environmental policies for all actors. Beverly Sauer's scholarship on risk rhetorics and feminist studies is grounded in the argument that risk studies are socially situated, and, as such, power structures embedded in technical communication about risk might explicitly or implicitly "silence the voices of women and others in matters of science and technology"; Sauer argues that these "voices" might have important insights to offer to risk deliberation (2003, p. 4–5). This concern for both acknowledgment of science claims about complex and uncertain risks, and participatory opportunities to build constructs of risk are a major concern in my study as I explore public participant HVHF deliberation.

My study analyzes primary data to add to the body of research that looks beyond the notion of the "expert scientist" to assess risk related to energy policy and public participants by looking closely at an extended "authority" within public participation. For several decades, scholars have called for participatory input into environmental decisions that involve risk. These calls include institutional sponsors such as the National Research Council to engage the National Science Foundation and EPA for more participatory communicative research (Dietz and Stern, 2008, p. 4). But even with a call for more participation in deliberative spaces, there are questions about how public participants actually become a part of decision-making or take part in constructions of environmental risk due to a lack of integration of knowledge claims from varied participants. While there has been an acknowledgment of public participation in environmental issues and policy formation, the actual *process* of enacting different stakeholders is fraught with tension as varying interests informed by varying ideologies make knowledge claims and contest the authority to those claims. As such, the specific ways in which stakeholders might "deliberate" about environmental concern in the public sphere is both an important consideration in my research and situates my research within the emerging scholarship of environmental discourse scholarship as an empirical study about participant navigation of public space in an attempt to represent environmental risk. This is of particular concern when participants feel that discourses through which they must discuss risk are destructive or are perceived as coercive in that they destroy ecological destruction (2016, p. 24).

Norman Fairclough argues that discourses emerge from and maintain social, political, and cultural conditions (1989). Fairclough is clear about the ways in which language acts "as a form of social practice." (p. 22). Fairclough's notions of language embedded within society and language as a "socially conditioned process" (1989, p. 22) underscore the ways I approach language in this study. Fairclough points to the social aspects of "linguistic phenomena": "whenever speak, or listen or write or read, they do so in ways which are determined socially and have social effects" (p. 23). Similarly, Fairclough describes the ways in which "social phenomena are linguistic" by explaining that "language activity which goes on in social contexts (as all language activity does) is not merely a reflection or expression of social processes and practices, it is a *part* of those processes and practices" (p. 23). As such, understanding CDA as both a theory of discourse and social practice is particularly important to my study in terms of how language not only frames but directs HVHF deliberation. The language embedded in environmental risk participatory mechanisms that public participants navigated in my study points to ways in which participants might (or might not) deliberate about environmental risks. Time and time again, participants found that they did not have individual or even group agency to create meaning about environmental risk—they must, to borrow Fairclough's language, "speak, or listen or write or read" within socially constructed processes and practices that, many participants felt, did not represent their interests, or reflect long-term interests of the environment. In my study, I contend that interrogating participatory texts, processes, and practices at the linguistic level reveals deeply seated issues of power that actors must navigate in order to disrupt existing power structures. Fairclough's work extends to ways in which class, power, and capitalist economic systems sustain hegemony. The mechanisms that maintain these powerful systems are often "exercised in discourse" through ideologies that can facilitate "consent" (1989, p. 33). Fairclough and Fairclough (2015) argue that institutions that support HVHF create socially constructed institutional "constraints" for stakeholders within energy deliberations.

Similarly, Blommaert and Bulcaen's (2000) overview of CDA includes a discussion of "discourse-as-social-practice." To foreground "discourse-as-social-practice," Blommaert and Bulcaen point to "discourse–as-discursive-practice" to outline the ways in which semiotic systems, or text types, might be "produced, circulated, distributed, consumed" in a society (p. 449). Further, these scholars argue that issues of power and hegemonic constructs are maintained through social-discursive "consent." In other words, social meanings are shaped through dominant discourses that maintain powerful interests; I discuss this concern in more detail in the "procedural justice" portion of the literacy literature review later in this chapter. Blommaert and Bulcaen note an "interventionism," or commitment to "change" and "empowerment" that has emerged in some CDA scholarship, implying praxis as a possibility for CDA: "CDA advocates interventionism in the social practices it critically investigates" (p. 450).

In regards to the issue of consent, several CDA practitioners have focused on issues of the opacity of powerful neoliberal discourse that manufacture consent or legitimize particular value systems within institutions (Hasan, 2003; Fairclough, 2003; Blommaert, 2003). Holborrow defines neoliberal discourses as the way in which ideology, moving through the medium of a "sign" (language) manifests into apparent "natural truths," which serve to sustain constructed "common sense" ideologies that are increasingly sympathetic to global capitalism (2006). CDA, then, contributes to environmental justice frameworks I use in my research to critique neoliberal frames in environmental risk analysis.

In situating this study within a discourse framework, I turn to research focused on environmental discourse as indicated by the references to environmental communication and discourse scholars. While environmental discourse scholarship may not be explicitly part of CDA scholarship, environmental discourse scholarship and CDA scholarship are compatible in terms of examining issues of language, power, and resulting policy surrounding environmental issues.

In alignment with CDA scholarship, Dryzek (2005) points to the importance of analyzing language within environmental discourse: "this inquiry (environmental discourse) rests on the contention that language matters, that the way we construct, interpret, discuss, and analyze environmental problems has all kinds of consequences" (p. 10), particularly in terms of contested "deliberations" that result in policy or framework that maintains agency in policy or practice. Similarly, environmental discourse scholars Hajer and Versteeg (2005) refer to social constructions of language and context, most notably in terms of the limits language can place on the possibility of participating in a given social activity. This understanding of environmental discourse relates to CDA's inquisition into the ways in which language in practice within social constructs: "Language is not a neutral messenger of given interests and preferences, but it influences their very formation. Moreover, it enables and limits the range of practices and interactions in which actors can engage" (p. 166). In particular, Hajer and Versteeg cite the importance of discourse scholarship in investigating the "complex interactions" of environmental policy-making: "Concepts, such as sustainable development or the precautionary principle, are not and simply cannot be imposed in a top-down way, but are continually contested in a struggle about their meaning, interpretation and implementation." (2005, p. 176). In particular, Hajer and Versteeg show that discourse analysis reveals facets of deliberation: "In trying to make sense of this struggle, discourse analysis has three particular strengths: the capacity to reveal the role of language in politics, to reveal the embeddedness of language in practice and to illuminate mechanisms and answer 'how questions'" (2005, p. 176).

Environmental discourse scholarship is compatible with CDA in that both investigate language to reveal how power affects issues in environmental discourse by identifying contextual considerations. Hajer suggests that understanding the institutional contexts in which words are produced and circulated helps us to understand the socially constructed nature of discourse:

> developments in environmental politics critically depend on the specific social construction of environmental problems. We do not simply analyse what is being said, but also include the institutional context in which this is done and which co-determines what can be said meaningfully. (1995, p. 5)

NEOLIBERALISM AND HVHF DISCOURSE

To address the way in which consent happens linguistically, CDA scholarship more clearly theorizes the "legitimation" of power found in texts or mechanisms navigated by participants. For example, discourse structures position information that directs users to normative conclusions about content in texts (van Dijk, 2003, p. 358; van Leeuwen, 2007, p. 92). I argue, based on my data, a pro-industry frame is normalized within institutional tools. For example, Frank Fischer (2000), an environmental communications scholar, explicates how the framing of neopositivist strategies used by chosen experts empowers and creates legitimacy for experts and disempowers public deliberation opportunities about contested environmental claims:

> Because of the fundamental differences in the legitimacy and power of their respective languages—technical vs. everyday language—the interaction between the technocratic planners and the members of the local community tends to give shape to an unequal communicative relationship. . . . Such characterizations capture a belief in the superiority of scientific policy methods over political decision processes. (p. 18)

In my study, I focus on the CDA analytic lens of legitimation to explore language that contributes to the consolidation of power that occurs through managerial approaches (van Dijk, 2003, p. 360). To expand this notion of managerialism, I turn to environmental discourse scholars who point to problematic relationships between a managerial approach and power in terms of environmental "management" (Dryzek, 2005, p. 75). My focus on the legitimization of managerial approaches is largely applied to permitting *for* HVHF activity. I assert that language shapes public participant's orientations toward any deliberation about HVHF. For example, overwhelmingly, the ODNR, as denoted in its name, "Ohio Department of Natural *Resources*" represents nature as a resource—something that ultimately can be managed. According to my participants, institutions adopt attitudes that place a value on management of resources to capitalize on profits. The legitimation of this neoliberal framework occurs through the use and normalization of language frames that position the HVHF industry as "legitimate" though HVHF risk often has yet to be defined, tested, and regulated. Frustrations occur when participants find that they must deliberate about HVHF risk within a framework (such as ODNR public participatory tools) that is already positioned to allow HVHF activity. Environmental communications scholar Robert Fletcher points to CDA scholar Lemke who argues that neoliberalism is a "political project that endeavours to create a social reality that it suggests already exists" (qtd. in Fletcher, 2010, p. 173). In the case of my study, the emerging HVHF industry is often legitimized before its risks are fully understood or deliberated, largely through projections of what HVHF offers economically.

Within environmental discourse studies, the role of legitimation of certain ideologies to inform policy is largely seen as understudied (Steffek, 2009; Breeze, 2012). Environmental discourse scholar Steffek (2009) suggests that discourse scholars might attempt to "[Disentangle] the nexus of science, knowledge and politics" by turning to legitimation as a critical evaluation tool to understand environmental policy concerns, specifically focusing on "the *legitimation* of the institutions of environmental governance, their goals, policies, and procedures, through discursive processes" (p. 313). Here, Steffek explores the legitimation of environmental discourse framed by "expert" actors and the ways by which such discourses "might become exposed to wider public scrutiny" (p. 317).

Similarly, Breeze points to the ways in which legitimation of the oil and gas industry functions to maintain or create institutional agency through discourse through: "Legitimation aims to create an ideological space within which the institution can operate, enjoying sufficient social acceptance to pursue its activities freely" (2012, p. 4). Breeze outlines specifics of how this legitimation occurs: "Their discursive actions can thus be said to be ideological in nature, asserting the rightness of the institution's actions, preempting criticism from other social players and marking out the boundaries of the institution's rights and obligations within society" (2012, p. 4).

Breeze, in analyzing oil companies' responses after the 2010 Deepwater Horizon oil spill, contends that institutions create messages "which are intended to generate a positive evaluation and public image, combining classical promotional elements (self praise, positive connotations) with aspects of explanation and self-defence designed to pre-empt or defuse criticism on concrete issues (Malavasi, 2010)" (p. 5).

This attention to "institutional" legitimation and the ways in which institutions position themselves to legitimate various aspects of the HVHF industry is key to my research. I analyze, in this research, the ways in which participants question the legitimation practices of environmental institutions that "pre-empt" possibilities of environmental harm through managerial frames. Both Breeze and Seffek focus case studies on legitimation techniques used by institutions after an environmental accident, such as Breeze's investigations of legitimation attempts by looking at texts created by oil companies after the Deepwater Horizon oil spill. My research adds to this existing legitimation research about environmental discourse in that I explore participant responses as well as the institutional texts they must use prior to an environmental catastrophe. I look at the texts created by institutions legitimizing an industry (HVHF) operating on many complex uncertainties across time scales versus legitimation that occurs *after* an environmental disaster.

DISCOURSE LEGITIMATION PATTERNS

Legitimation occurs by invoking particular ideologies, so it is important in my research to discuss discourse scholars who trace the way different actors define complex environmental risks (if they define a particular issue as a risk at all) through value systems inherent in environmental ideologies. Several scholars discuss types of environmental discourse ideologies that inform knowledge making and environmental risk framing: Hajer (1995), Lash, Szerszynski, and Wynne (1996), Harvey (1999), Dryzek (2005), and Feindt and Oels (2005). My work more clearly focuses on issues of the ways in which neoliberal values are often framed through institutional risk participatory mechanisms which public participants must access in order to enter HVHF deliberation. These varied environmental ideologies are important to consider in terms of distinct neoliberal issues as revealed by CDA and environmental discourse scholarship. Capitalist discursive frames might frame environmental risk very differently than other discursive frames. Environmental discourse scholars contend that current energy policies in the United States are positioned to legitimize "development" or "industry" frames (Dryzek, 2005). In the industry frame, environmental risks emerge and are dealt with in response to inevitable industry development. This is in opposition to a precautionary frame, which urges precaution in terms of what an industry can or should do. Similarly, environmental discourse scholar Harvey explores the notion of a "standard view" of environmental policy as a type of "environmental management" which ultimately supports existing extractive and production practices promoting "business as usual" capitalist economic systems (1999).

An investigation of "standard view" discourses can be tied to rhetorical considerations. Environmental rhetoricians Killingsworth and Palmer (1992) discuss how deliberative tools and literate practices citizens can use to participate in environmental risk policy are limited. These institutionally sponsored literate practices (ways of reading and writing) create institutional agency by orchestrating "instrumental documents" which act as "steering mechanisms" to achieve social solidarity that maintains a hierarchy of environmental policy invested in such a standard view (p. 166). Such mechanisms, then, favor particular energy policies. They create the opportunity for one discourse to appear as a "natural" social consensus, without having to attend to alternative narratives. This phenomena of an orchestrated consensus is clear in Curran's work on discourse narratives and the difficulty in establishing wind energy systems in Australia: "a discourse is strengthened by its capacity to 'naturalise' its meanings . . . in short, when particular narrative positions advanced appear to derive 'naturally' from a social consensus about values and socio-economic priorities" (2012, p. 243).

Concerns of power and agency and environmental risk are compounded by unequal access to risk reporting tools and the ways these tools are used by different agents. Of particular concern in this study, then, are moments when discursively constructed literacy practices tend to guide a premeditated outcome, one that stymies alternative discussions, such as renewable energy development, or does not fully represent the risks inherent in unconventional fossil fuel production.

However, competing discursive frames can challenge what Simmons terms as "pseudoparticipation" of citizens in deliberations about environmental policy (2007, p. 38) that "normalize" an "inevitable" future as framed by dominant discourses (Hajer, 1995; Dryzek, 2005). Environmental justice frameworks, for example, challenge "industry" or "standard" ideologies due to a concern with "the legacy of a disproportionate burden imposed on poor and minority communities by environmental harmful conditions, [and calls for] more inclusive opportunities for those who are most affected to be heard in the decisions made by public agencies" (Cox, 2006, p. 290).

CASE STUDY: PRO-HVHF STORYLINES WITHIN ENVIRONMENTAL RISK

My research enters into discussions with scholars who point to the increasing need to critically examine the current literate and communicative practices concerning environmental risks.

Rhetorical Analysis Methods: Is/Ought Constructions and Stasis

My investigation explores coding schemes that seek patterns in rhetoric or the "available means of persuasion" (Cox, 2006, p. 53), an important consideration in terms of how citizens use literacy practices to navigate and participate in public deliberations about environmental risk and energy policy. I ground my work in notions of socially constructed rhetorics of risk as explored in the literature review, for example, Sauer's extension of traditional Aristotelian rhetorics to include both "postmodern and feminist awareness" (2003, p. 5) account for socially constructed notions of risk and those who are able to discuss risk at all. In Sauer's words, this means "that existing communication practices within industries are shaped and constrained by political and economic assumptions that may inadvertently silence or render invisible the kinds of information that decision makers need to assess and manage risk in hazardous environments" (2003, p. 5). Additionally, Grabill and Simmon's "critical rhetoric of risk communication" (1998, p. 429) explores more deeply who is included in deliberations about risk communication beyond "experts" who simply disseminate information in a linear fashion to a passive lay person audience. It was important for me, in the research design and collection process, to allow participants to detail patterns as they emerged through participant use of environmental risk participatory mechanisms. While I had noted patterns of participant frustration in linear communication patterns from my pilot data, I wanted to give participants the opening to express how this impacted them in use. As such, I approached my data collection informed by the tenets of Grounded Theory where I gathered data from participants after which I coded for rhetorical patterns (Glaser and Straus, 1967). I entered into rhetorical analysis with a plan to understand issues of authority and environmental policy implementation, and I reexamined patterns as they emerged from participant discussion, participant analysis of a text or procedure, or my own analysis of a text or procedure that a participant referred to.

In my research, a major concern about risk communication for all eighteen participants was the way in which deliberation about an environmental risk might simply not occur at all—that publics are simply not engaged in a deliberation about environmental risk. Through my pilot and dissertation research, I found rhetorical patterns that include tensions about the authority of who is deemed worthy of entering a deliberation. Often, there is little inquiry into investigating values underlying environmental risk policies (often portrayed as based in "science," which activists pressed to reveal more nuances . . . *whose* science?) I found patterns in Schiappa's "is/ought" rhetorical construction, which might uncover notions of rhetorical authority in terms of who can make risk policy formation or who might invoke the is/ought construction. Who determines what *is,* a definitional concern, and what *ought* to be, a sociopolitical concern? (Schiappa, 2003). Schiappa speaks to definitional concerns in terms of rhetorical analysis "A rhetorical analysis of definition, then, investigates how people persuade other people to adopt and use certain definitions to the exclusion of others" (1998, p. 2). Of considerable concern in my study is the authority by which one might be able to make definitions used in risk policy. This is/ought distinction, as connected to authority, dovetails neatly into the work of Fahnestock and Secor (1985), who suggest application of the stasis, or levels of questions to clarify points and consider assumptions, as a possible deliberative tool for risk stakeholders. This fit well into another major concern of all eighteen participants. Participants regularly discussed disparate policy implementation of the emerging HVHF industry across different states. Participants in Ohio and Pennsylvania, in particular, were often frustrated by the lack of regulation that occurred at their state lines. Participants in New York often referred to Ohio and Pennsylvania HVHF as cautionary tales about the lack of regulation (there was a moratorium, then a ban on HVHF drilling activity in New York during my data collection process). In my rhetorical analysis, I found that participants could often NOT deliberate about HVHF risks because the authority of institutional reporting stymied discussion. If they could deliberate about HVHF risks, participants discussed systemic risk deliberation limitations in stasis, see table 2.1.

In my research, I also found patterns of the rhetorical notion of stasis (Fahnestock and Secor, 1985) were helpful to categorize disparate policies in various states. Questions of fact (*is* there risk?), questions of definition

Table 2.1 Rhetorical Analysis Coding Scheme

Rhetorical Analysis:

Can Public Participants Deliberate about HVHF Risks within Institutional Environmental Reporting Tools?

A. No, Deliberation Is Not Apparent or Stalls
By whose authority is deliberation stymied?

B. Yes, Deliberation Proceeds **Within** *Institutional Reporting; Participants Discuss Systemic Deliberation Limitations*

In what part of stasis does this deliberation occur? (Fahnestock and Secor, 1985, Schiappa, 2003)

1. *question of fact*
2. *question of definition* **(IS)**
3. *question of value*
4. *question of jurisdiction (policy)* **(OUGHT)**

By what authority (ethos) are these levels of stasis answered/maintained? (Schiappa, 2003)

(*what* is the risk?), questions of value (is it *important to do something* about this risk?), and questions of jurisdiction (what exactly *ought* to be done about the risk?) helped to clarify different approaches across states to HVHF risk. Simultaneously, I continue to interrogate the issue of authority within the stasis—I argue that it is important to understand by whose authority levels of stasis are invoked to clearly understand disparate risk representation across states. I expected and found patterns of value as various notions of "science" lay claim to varied policies, again, an issue of authority or ethos. Carolan notes that the issue of value in this scientific discussion is noteworthy: "That is, while these controversies may appear on the surface to rest on disputed questions of fact, beneath often reside differing positions of value; values that can give shape to differing understandings of what 'the facts' are." (2008, p. 734). Carolan further discusses the way in which "uncertainty" is always grounded in value, making the concept of "consensus" in these complicated discussions problematic. These issues of contested authority and stasis formulate a rhetorical critique of institutional risk reporting.

As I worked through my rhetorical analysis, I provided examples from public participant interviews or TAPs to showcase rhetorical patterns that emerge from the "no" and the "yes" responses when investigating *why deliberation did not occur* and *limitations to deliberation within environmental participatory mechanisms*. When applicable, I included commentary from participants themselves (from interviews and TAPs) about issues of authority and stasis constructs. However, I also further analyzed texts participants might have led me to, as participants were not rhetorical scholars and our interviews and TAPs were not designed for participants to perform a formal rhetorical analysis. It is from this participant-sourced data that I chose to conduct further analysis after noting discursive patterns across participant responses. A sample analysis from a participant screenshot from "Peg" is included in figure 2.1.

Generally, across participant TAPs and interviews, I found the following patterns in risk deliberation difficulties.

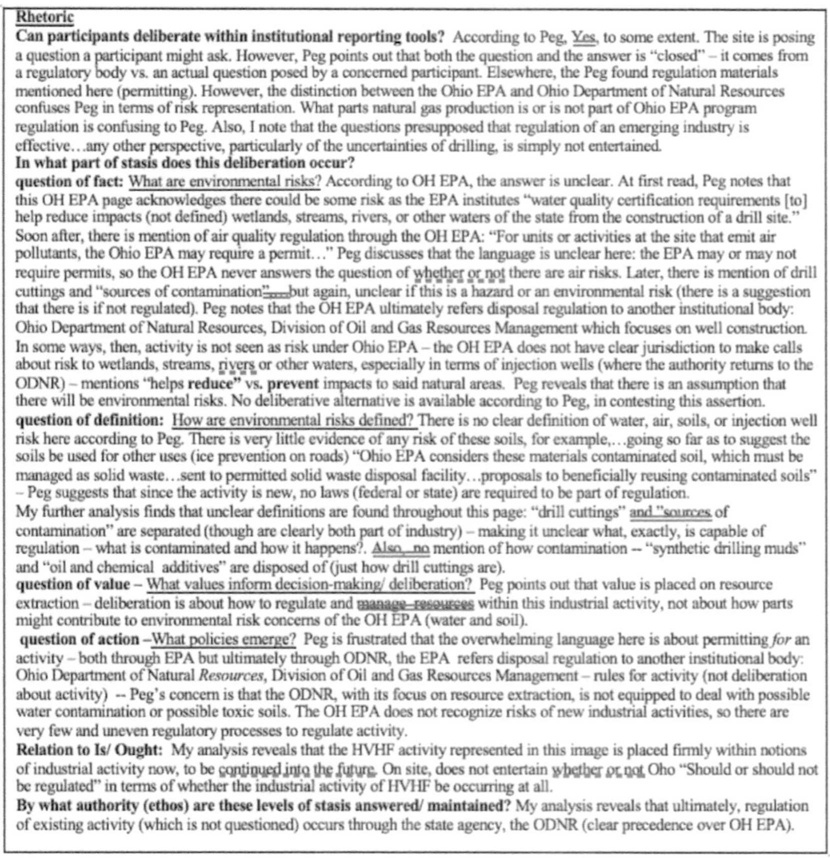
Rhetoric

Can participants deliberate within institutional reporting tools? According to Peg, Yes, to some extent. The site is posing a question a participant might ask. However, Peg points out that both the question and the answer is "closed" – it comes from a regulatory body vs. an actual question posed by a concerned participant. Elsewhere, the Peg found regulation materials mentioned here (permitting). However, the distinction between the Ohio EPA and Ohio Department of Natural Resources confuses Peg in terms of risk representation. What parts natural gas production is or is not part of Ohio EPA program regulation is confusing to Peg. Also, I note that the questions presupposed that regulation of an emerging industry is effective…any other perspective, particularly of the uncertainties of drilling, is simply not entertained.

In what part of stasis does this deliberation occur?

question of fact: What are environmental risks? According to OH EPA, the answer is unclear. At first read, Peg notes that this OH EPA page acknowledges there could be some risk as the EPA institutes "water quality certification requirements [to] help reduce impacts (not defined) wetlands, streams, rivers, or other waters of the state from the construction of a drill site." Soon after, there is mention of air quality regulation through the OH EPA: "For units or activities at the site that emit air pollutants, the Ohio EPA may require a permit…" Peg discusses that the language is unclear here: the EPA may or may not require permits, so the OH EPA never answers the question of whether or not there are air risks. Later, there is mention of drill cuttings and "sources of contamination"…but again, unclear if this is a hazard or an environmental risk (there is a suggestion that there is if not regulated). Peg notes that the OH EPA ultimately refers disposal regulation to another institutional body: Ohio Department of Natural Resources, Division of Oil and Gas Resources Management which focuses on well construction. In some ways, then, activity is not seen as risk under Ohio EPA – the OH EPA does not have clear jurisdiction to make calls about risk to wetlands, streams, rivers or other waters, especially in terms of injection wells (where the authority returns to the ODNR) – mentions "helps **reduce"** vs. **prevent** impacts to said natural areas. Peg reveals that there is an assumption that there will be environmental risks. No deliberative alternative is available according to Peg, in contesting this assertion.

question of definition: How are environmental risks defined? There is no clear definition of water, air, soils, or injection well risk here according to Peg. There is very little evidence of any risk of these soils, for example,…going so far as to suggest the soils be used for other uses (ice prevention on roads) "Ohio EPA considers these materials contaminated soil, which must be managed as solid waste…sent to permitted solid waste disposal facility…proposals to beneficially reusing contaminated soils" – Peg suggests that since the activity is new, no laws (federal or state) are required to be part of regulation.

My further analysis finds that unclear definitions are found throughout this page: "drill cuttings" and "sources of contamination" are separated (though are clearly both part of industry) – making it unclear what, exactly, is capable of regulation – what is contaminated and how it happens?. Also, no mention of how contamination -- "synthetic drilling muds" and "oil and chemical additives" are disposed of (just how drill cuttings are).

question of value – What values inform decision-making/ deliberation? Peg points out that value is placed on resource extraction – deliberation is about how to regulate and ~~manage resources~~ within this industrial activity, not about how parts might contribute to environmental risk concerns of the OH EPA (water and soil).

question of action –What policies emerge? Peg is frustrated that the overwhelming language here is about permitting *for* an activity – both through EPA but ultimately through ODNR, the EPA refers disposal regulation to another institutional body: Ohio Department of Natural *Resources*, Division of Oil and Gas Resources Management – rules for activity (not deliberation about activity) -- Peg's concern is that the ODNR, with its focus on resource extraction, is not equipped to deal with possible water contamination or possible toxic soils. The OH EPA does not recognize risks of new industrial activities, so there are very few and uneven regulatory processes to regulate activity.

Relation to Is/ Ought: My analysis reveals that the HVHF activity represented in this image is placed firmly within notions of industrial activity now, to be continued into the future. On site, does not entertain whether or not Oho "Should or should not be regulated" in terms of whether the industrial activity of HVHF be occurring at all.

By what authority (ethos) are these levels of stasis answered/ maintained? My analysis reveals that ultimately, regulation of existing activity (which is not questioned) occurs through the state agency, the ODNR (clear precedence over OH EPA).

Figure 2.1 Representative Sample, Peg's TAP, Rhetorical Analysis Coding. *Source*: Screenshot by author.

Lack of Access to Public Meetings

- No advertising of upcoming public meetings about risk related to HVHF (including on local, municipal calendars).
- Difficulty finding upcoming meetings on institutional websites, like the Ohio Department of Natural Resources, PA Department of Environmental Protection, and the New York Department of Environmental Conservation.
- A concern of lack of institutional protocol to field risk questions: questions to the ODNR would be sent to the Ohio EPA which, in turn, was sent back to the ODNR.
- If advertising a meeting, too short a time period for participants to make plans to attend local meetings related to HVHF.

No public meetings before the industry commenced—informational meetings about the inevitable HVHF processing plant were noted by several activists in Pennsylvania and Ohio.

Lack of Access within Public Meetings

- Planned industry representative speakers at initial informational meetings positioned the industry as "inevitable," and discussion of banning the industry or parts of industry by stakeholders as unreasonable.
- Not allowing certain public participants to speak.
- Sifting through public comments on index cards to choose what public comment to respond to, carefully choosing which questions to ask the ODNR or PA DEP representative invited to speak to the public.
- Obstructing recording of public meetings.
- Limiting the time in which public participants can speak.
- Framing those who speak against oil and gas as "disruptive."
- Intimidation: Representatives from pro-industry groups recasting meetings (Energy In Depth, PR group), including personal attacks on activists.

Lack of Access on Institutional Sites

Additionally, participants found patterns of difficulty in assessing risk on several institutional websites.

1. Difficulty in Finding Details of HVHF Operation Information.
    A. Access to Physical Public Meetings.
    B. Access to Deliberation in Public Meetings.
    C. Accessible Language on Official Online Sites.
    D. Access to Online Mapping on Official Online Sites.

2. Top-down Explanations Suggesting No Risk or Manageable Risk.
3. Pseudo and Superficial Participation.
4. Time and Money; Permit and Public Records Requests.

Some of the issues outlined above are explored with participant data below.

Lack of Accessible Mapping

Ohio

Oil and gas well locators that might help participants find oil and gas activity in their vicinity, according to participants, were extremely difficult to use. One must know the names of the well and navigate highly technical "layers" for sites, and the maps do not provide much information about unknown well sites. This led Kim to muse, "So you must know the well to find the well. That doesn't help me to see wells I don't know about." Keys did not match images, wait times to find well information were quite long, and the language was very highly technical.

Peg found the navigation to be onerous: "This would take [a public user] forever and [as a public user] I would give up immediately because it isn't really what you would call user friendly." Peg identified a well with highly technical geological information versus using more accessible mapping identifiers that are common on basic Google mapping programs. The second sequence was Peg's attempt to find a well by searching for its name; this navigation was highly technical, and the information about the well name was not easily available on a mapping site or other parts of the ODNR site. The third sequence in the series revealed some directional drilling on each of the well pads, but Peg noted that the directional arrows that stem from each well aren't fully explained. This is a concern for a homeowner who might be worried about lateral drilling. In response to a highly publicized well that had been shut down due to seismic activities, "When they tell you they shut down a well, they just shut down one little [direction]."

Peg found that clicking on the "information pop up" from the bottom right of the third map in the sequence did not provide information that a concerned public participant might be seeking.

When Peg clicked the "Information Popup" tab, she did find some information about the well, but that information was highly technical and concerned with outputs rather than her concerns about the chemicals involved in the operation, the waterways that might be impacted by the operation, and the air quality impacted by the operation. Perhaps Peg's experience is most succinctly summed by her comment "This is a hideous site [for accessing well information] . . . I gave up over and over again . . . . I don't usually bother with ODNR because I know they are a bunch of corrupt bastards." Peg could not clearly find HVHF risk information at the culmination of her search.

Pennsylvania

In PA, such obfuscation occurs in different ways. For example, Shelly explained that in order to access online gas mapping information, stakeholders must navigate to the oil and gas reports, which are situated in the Business and Energy tab through the Pennsylvania Department of Environmental Protection. In order to access the oil and gas reports, one must install Silverlight programming. Shelly noted that participants might be turned off from doing so because they simply don't know how to install such programming and fear computer viruses, "For people who have Macs, that's less of a worry because the risk of getting a virus is less, but most people have PCs, especially in the areas where fracking is going on because they are lower economic areas." Thus, access to technology to navigate institutional sites was a concern of participants.

Additionally, participants found stasis issues in terms of discussing the following risks—which were defined differently across states: contamination risks, radioactive risks, seismic risks, injection well risks, landowner property risks, health risks, and global climate change risks.

Time and Money; Permitting and Public Records Requests

Ohio

One constraint reported by many participants attempting to navigate HVHF was the positioning of public participants to have to contest HVHF industry permits in Ohio and Pennsylvania. In other words, public participants could not assume that environmental regulatory bodies would seek HVHF risk for them. Diane reported the small amount of time participants had to submit a challenge to an HVHF permit that might impact one's property:

> Craziness, do you know that you only have 30 days from the time you find out about an issue until you have to put this [challenge] together. It was day and night . . . it was a cram session . . . hours of (research) . . . I earned a master's degree in fracking in a period of a month . . . it was crazy.

Here, Diane makes an assertion that she must find the burden of proof of HVHF risk within a deliberative system that offers her little time and few tools to do so.

Several participants in Ohio, including Kim, stressed that across the board, time frames for oil and gas permitting have been lessened considerably through House Bill 8 to promote permitting activity, which lessened time for participants to gather information about HFHV risks and find the proper "window" to make public comment to the regulatory body about well and drilling plans: "HB 8 is supposed to make . . . the length of time shorter so that if somebody says they want to drill . . . it is all supposed to happen a lot easier . . . Ohio HB 8 is just another law that puts corporate rights above human rights or above people's rights." Kim continued to express her frustration with the length of time a public participant could contest a permit by pointing to property values: "If you were an unwilling property owner, they're trying to pool . . . to get enough property to do a fracking [operation] you only have forty-five days . . . to get legal representation to fight this . . . you don't have enough time to put this house on the market."

This pattern of reduced public comment time is similar in Pennsylvania and New York. Interestingly, Kim found that the same expediency in applying for a ban on HVHF activity was simply not considered, including stipulations for "completing" a ban application, with significant possible procedural time constraints.

Across the board, participants in my study noted very long wait periods to hear back from the ODNR or the DEP about environmental risk inquiries, including public records requests. Peg felt these wait times were intentional: "If you frustrate someone long enough, they will give up. You can't wait for two years to find out that something is harming you."

This concern about the burden of proof regarding time and money was echoed by Nancy, who spent money on getting baseline water testing near her home when HVHF activity commenced nearby: "[It was] money out of my pocket. 344 out of my pocket." According to Nancy, an option for free baseline water testing was completed through a water company that had known links to the HVHF industry, an option Nancy rejected.

Three participants in Ohio, Peg, Val, and Craig, who could not access information at the state level, navigated requests for Freedom of Information Act through the federal EPA. As noted earlier, this process is very expensive, while the others were able to raise funds through activist community groups to which they belonged. One had to hire a lawyer and pay a fee to access the information. Of the three who filed a request for information through the Freedom of Information Act, many found that such recourse was not accessible to general users, particularly those without computers. Craig reported: "The Freedom of Information Act requests frequently costs a lot of money . . . hundreds of dollars."

Pennsylvania

Diane also paid a fee to access state records in Pennsylvania, detailing a trip to Harrisburg, a drive of several hours. Once she paid her fee, finding information about wells near her home was still difficult:

> You have to know exactly what you want and you have to fill out all of this information. The very first one that I did . . . there was a room full of records . . . and we had know idea . . . what we were looking for. We stumbled onto that well packet by accident . . . we asked for things that we didn't know what they were. Not only is this difficult to navigate, you don't know what you want or what it is housed in. It is almost as though they purposefully make it difficult so you can't find it.

Diane's quandary shows the way in which institutional framing of risk information is perceived by public participants.

STASIS

Finally, there are several areas of stasis where HVHF risk was found to be stymied. In these examples, participants from different states worked through definitions of fact, definition, value, and jurisdiction (policy) differently. Overall, my research revealed inequities across states in representing risk.

Stasis 1: HVHF Drilling Chemical Risks

A concern reported by many participants is the components of HVHF chemicals. New York banned HVHF drilling in part due to questions about uncertainties about possible chemical contamination. While Ohio and Pennsylvania provided chemical disclosure, such disclosure was very limited and largely allowed HVHF activity. Both Pennsylvania and Ohio state agencies regulate chemicals through the Pennsylvania Department of Environmental Protection or the Ohio Department of Natural Resources. A stasis analysis shows that while HVHF chemical risks may be acknowledged in Pennsylvania and Ohio, the definitions of risks are vague and are represented as manageable through regulations. An "is" inquiry reveals that chemical risks do exist across all three states. An "ought" inquiry about what to do about the risks differs among states, as New York bans HVHF drilling while Pennsylvania and Ohio attempt to regulate chemicals, revealing uneven risk distribution.

Participants had serious reservations about the ability of state regulatory institutions to effectively regulate drilling chemicals in states whose value systems allow for minimal disclosure of chemical components to protect company "trade secrets" and whose jurisdictions allow for HVHF drilling. This was very clear in the way in which participants might access chemical disclosure information for emergencies or to understand chemicals used in drilling activity near their homes.

Ohio

For example, only one of the six participants in Ohio, Craig, knew how to navigate to the chemical disclosure page provided by the ODNR. Though there are some ways to navigate to chemical components of HVHF drilling activity, such navigation was difficult. Craig's TAP revealed the limitations of chemical disclosure on the ODNR site and calls into question Ohio's construction of chemical risk through definition (is) and the Ohio policy protections (or lack of protections) related to chemical risks (ought).

First, Craig noted that the ODNR regulates chemical disclosure rather than either the federal or the Ohio EPA, a decision that occurred long before HVHF activity was practiced at the scale it is practiced now: "The ODNR applied for and received authority over injection wells from the EPA in 1983, so there is no reason to go to the U.S. EPA website." As the ODNR is often viewed as friendly to HVHF activity, Craig noted the gaps in ODNR accountability, "They [US EPA] are supposed to audit the ODNR's injection well program every few years—but you can't find that on here. You have to make a records request." As public records requests cost hundreds of dollars, this cost creates a stumbling block for public participants seeking information about the safety of injection wells near their homes. Craig went on to describe the limitations in terms of value systems embedded in the chemical disclosure process found on the ODNR sites and how that compromised community safety: "Fracfocus is industry run . . . we wrote a report about how Fracfocus didn't disclose all of the chemicals that the U.S. EPA found on the Eisenbarth well fire . . . that happened last year."

Craig noted that emergency information related to chemical incidents is very difficult to navigate, which should concern both firefighters and health officials who would have a very hard time finding the chemical components of a particular spill. Chemical components can be found only after a series of difficult navigations.

Craig, who had a chemistry background, also found chemical components to be listed in fragmented form, obscuring how much of a chemical might be used, and whether that chemical, especially in conjunction with other chemicals, might be harmful to the environment (plants, animals, waterways) or humans. "Notice that they don't have the actual amounts of the chemical. They have these unhelpful percentage . . . 'the maximum ingredient concentration in hydrofracking fluid percent by mass' . . . they don't give you the total mass of the fracking fluid so you can't figure out the mass of the chemical . . ."

To find more information about possible chemical contamination in Ohio, Craig pointed out that, once again, one must apply for a Freedom of Information Act request, which costs hundreds of dollars and takes quite a bit of time.

Pennsylvania

Pennsylvania participants were particularly troubled by the limitations of disclosure, which they felt honored industry (in the form of trade secrets) over human health through PA Act thirteen, which made it difficult for doctors and health professionals to obtain information about oil and gas chemicals to treat patients who may have come into contact with these chemicals due to HVHF. The reasoning involves the value placed on the "trade secrets" of the HVHF chemical components, as defined by the oil and gas industry (Woodall, 2016).

Stasis II: HVHF Drilling Contamination Risks—Water and Soil

Another major concern participants noted was issues of accessing regulatory risk tools to understand possible water and soil contamination due to HVHF activity. A stasis analysis reveals different water and soil policies that varied across New York, Pennsylvania, and Ohio, showing unequal risk distribution.

Participants found definitional variations (the "is") in water and soil protections that led to differing policies (the "ought") among states. When water and soil risk was minimized through institutional representations, policies to protect water or soil were weakened or were non-existent. These policies in response to contamination risks varied by location (see table 2.2).

As a representative sample, I show Ohio participants who felt that the Ohio EPA, which posts the following mission on its website: "Protect human health and the environment by characterizing and protecting groundwater quality and ensuring that Ohio's public water systems provide adequate supplies of safe drinking water," could be a place where participants could access possible soil or water contamination. However, several participants were dissatisfied with the way in which the Ohio EPA did not apply water protection in risk deliberation related to HVHF.

The Ohio EPA, Peg noted, distanced itself considerably from any involvement with making decisions about oil and gas industry activities that might involve water, even though "clean water" is a clear concern of the Ohio EPA (the two sites, ODNR and Ohio EPA, link to each other). Here, the definitional concerns of "water protection," an "is" concern, as practiced by the EPA, do not apply to broad portions of HVHF water regulation, suggesting to participants that water protection is only valued in scenarios that do not infringe upon HVHF activity. Because the ODNR, a group that regularly provides permits for HVHF activity, has the final say in whether HVHF might harm water, Ohio participants felt that the Ohio EPA could not follow up on water protection programs in place prior to widespread HVHF activity. Peg observed, "The ODNR has primacy" as she browsed the site. Participants reported that the HVHF industry uses high volumes of water in the production, transportation, and disposal processes of HVHF, so participants found the way in which water protection policy and HVHF are not represented on the Ohio EPA to be significant. Peg pointed out that as the Ohio EPA does *not* consider HVHF water contamination under its jurisdiction, and HVHF is not obligated to abide by the Clean Water Act, the risk of fracking fluid in water is a very real concern for participants. She was upset reading over a Source Water Protection Plan developed by the Ohio EPA that ignores HVHF activity.

> Yes, there is a Source Water Protection Plan . . . and they [the Ohio EPA] are ignoring it; this is really insulting crap. This is nuts . . . it's a whole bunch of stuff that isn't relevant to people who are hit by this industry [HVHF]. It's a whole bunch of stuff that makes you think . . . maybe this will help me . . . Fracking is exempt from the Safe Drinking Water Act . . . Under the Clean Water Act, fracking gets a pass.

Thus, the water protection, as defined and touted by the Ohio EPA, is rendered largely ambiguous in terms of providing risk protection in regards to HVHF extraction and industry.

Similarly, the ways in which soil risk might not be represented as an HVHF under the jurisdiction of the Ohio EPA caused considerable concern among participants. Participants identified that the Ohio EPA appears to not regulate the issue of possible hazards to the soil, instead defining the drill cuttings as "contaminated soil" vs. hazardous waste (an "is" designation). Instead, the regulation of water risks is passed to the ODNR, which participants note does not have an extensive water protection program (an "ought" designation). The ways that water and soil contamination might be defined have resulted in various water and soil protection policies in New York, Pennsylvania, and Ohio (see table 2.2 at the end of this chapter).

Stasis III: Radioactivity

Several participants were concerned about radioactivity in many parts of HVHF production and disposal, but regulatory sites routinely denied risks—though they were not always clear about what part of the disposal was not radioactive. A stasis analysis clarifies how participants question the methods of defining radioactive waste. Participants were concerned about how states test (or do not test) to determine radioactivity within HVHF waste. Again, we see the "is" and "ought" through definitional and policy concerns as informed by values. In this section of the stasis, it is noted that all states do accept some drilling waste, but Ohio accepts more HVHF waste than either Pennsylvania or New York. This is partly because Ohio can accept waste through state regulatory measures, while Pennsylvania waste is subject to federal regulations (Kowalski, 2014).

Ohio

Several Ohio participants argued that much of the waste accepted in Ohio was not permitted to be disposed of across state lines in Pennsylvania, but there was no explanation as to why this was so. Largely because HVHF is not regulated federally, any radioactivity found is not part of the Comprehensive Environmental Response, Compensation, and Liability Act (CERCLA, commonly known as the Superfund Law), though none of these states are required to consistently test for radiation risk (Steinzor and Baizel, 2015, p. 21). Since testing is not a requirement, there are questions about what defines "harmful" radioactivity in disposal materials (an "is" concern). In essence, participants noted that the lack of consistent, binding protocols for the testing of the chemical constituents of raw and solidified waste prior to disposal could prove problematic for landfills, and in turn, for soil and water quality. As long as comprehensive chemical testing is not required, and landfills instead rely on such factors as appearance, passing the paint filter test (discussed below), and the general declarations of waste generators to determine how waste is managed and disposed of, the actual content of waste and its potential impacts are largely unknown (Steinzor and Baizel, 2015). A lack of testing leads to vagueness in the definition of radioactivity that results in policies that participants felt did not account for *possible* radioactive risks.

In Peg's exploration from the ODNR drill cuttings, for example, they are NOT currently considered to be hazardous waste because "state and federal regulations do not classify drill cuttings as hazardous waste." Peg found this policy decision to be both premature and disconcerting as widespread radioactivity tests had yet to be conducted (so there was an impasse about the definitional concern) and discussed worries about the effect of possible radioactivity on the health of participants who lived near HVHF disposal locations.

However, in neighboring states, participants also revealed uncertainties about the radioactive nature of wastes. Since the beginning of my data collection, despite language on institutional sites, several academic studies have pointed to radioactivity risks inherent in HVHF drill cuttings—various health and industry experts debate the findings in terms of human health consequences (Hurdle, 2015). My stasis analysis shows, more clearly, how states that accept more HVHF waste face possible radioactivity waste risk, regardless of how institutions position themselves as managers (see table 2.2 at the end of this chapter).

Stasis IV: Seismic Activity Risk

Many participants (myself included) experienced earthquakes in areas that accepted HVHF or fracking wastewater in injection wells.

Ohio

Seismic activity was particularly notable in Ohio, a state that routinely accepted HVHF waste as discussed in the previous section. However, Ohio participants felt representations or definitions of risk related to these events to be limited (an "is" concern). In a stasis analysis, the way seismic activities are defined and regulated (a policy or "ought" concern) shows the ways in which state institutions tend to downplay seismic risk, though Ohio, which accepts more HVHF wastewater, has experienced more seismic activity than Pennsylvania or New York.

Nancy found that risk as related to earthquakes is ascertained by the ODNR, but the course of action, which is essentially to recover resources, shows particular value orientations of resource recovery that result in policies favoring HVHF (an "ought" concern).

Also, Nancy and Peg were frustrated with the time it took to validate what they "felt"; science, such as seismology reports, takes years to complete, long after damage is done (several participants complained of or knew of home foundation damage due to HVHF). Nancy noted that the representation shows seismic activity as only *possible* vs. *likely*, and the representation continued to stress the way in which Ohio might regulate seismic activity related to HVHF though those "comprehensive regulatory" systems had clearly failed in light of several earthquakes occurring in the area. Also, the industry status quo is clear as areas that have been linked to earthquakes due to HVHF disposal will likely continue: "further hydraulic fracturing at the site is suspended but the company will be permitted to recover resources from five of the previously drilled wells located on the pad."

Nancy and Peg found that this seismic statement was an example of few or no places within ODNR regulatory risk reporting tools to find ways to discuss risks that have been acknowledged within institutional frameworks. In this case, the ODNR was slow in acknowledging the risks or engaging citizens about the seismic risk, before or after the event. There is very little information shared about potential risks of HVHF activities that still might cause similar events. The language on the ODNR site, according to participants, certainly suggests doubt that seismic activities were caused solely by hydraulic fracturing (an "is" concern) and suggests a policy that gives credence to regulation by experts vs. citizen deliberation about this issue (an "ought" concern). Meanwhile, both Nancy and Peg had collected academic research that directly related seismic activity to HVHF activity. All states' environmental regulatory institutions tended to downplay seismic risks through HVHF-related activity, but as Ohio regularly accepts more waste (that is largely untested), Ohio participants were keenly aware of a concentration of possible radioactive wastes in their state (see table 2.2 at the end of this section).

Stasis V: Injection Well Risks

Ohio

Injection wells, as mentioned in the previous "seismic" statement, are particularly prolific in Ohio. Because of this heavy concentration of injection wells in one state versus others, participants questioned possible risks associated with injection wells and varied definitions ("is" concerns) and policies ("ought" concerns) of injection well risks among states. A stasis analysis about injection well risk shows that injection well risks are positioned as minimal, and the number of injection wells varies across the states. An "is" inquiry reveals that states tend to view injection well risks as "minimal." An "ought" analysis reveals that Ohio, free of federal regulatory restrictions for such wells, moves forward with policies that allow for the bulk of Pennsylvania's wastewater to be transported to Ohio. Ohio is often framed as a sacrifice zone where social constructs lead to Ohio accepting disposal because of a marginalized identity as a result of past industry (George, 2016b). As such, Ohio disproportionately accepts more HVHF wastes by permitting more injection wells than neighboring states (Kowalski, 2014).

The acceptance of such wastes was of considerable concern among Ohio residents. Nancy's TAP reveals an ODNR site that. On the ODNR site, a statement presenting the reasoning for the placement of wells is stated in terms of economics:

> the location of any facility is a business decision . . . .It should be noted that oil and natural production and investment in the eastern portion of the state vastly outpaces the rest of the state as well. Economics dictate that disposal wells will be located near productions.

Nancy contended that the ODNR answers don't fully address the question and answers with an ideology that values economics and industry above curtailing possible environmental risk. It must be noted that it is not clear where the question, "Why doesn't ODNR limit the number of injection wells in a particular area . . . ?" comes from, or how many concerned citizens have asked this question. This economic ideology will be explored in more detail in the CDA portion of this study.

During a pilot study meeting, I attended public meetings in which concerned public participants in Northeast Ohio decried the large number of injection wells in NE Ohio, citing that most of the waste came from PA. At this point, an industry representative suggested that the geology of Eastern Ohio was more conducive to injection. Both PA and OH regulatory bodies claim that injection wells can be regulated safely . . . though PA limits the amount. There was an outcry at this point, as the Pennsylvania state line was only miles away, and citizens knew the geology was not much different within this short distance. Participants, instead, argued that the issue was a different perception of risk in each state.

Public participants in Ohio critiqued the extensive injection well permitting in the state, suggesting prospective risks due to the lack of regulation of injection wells. As Craig suggested, "There were four injection wells on the same property injecting into the same formation within a quarter of a mile from each other. It seemed like an idiotic thing to do." Craig questioned the lack of regulations on injection well construction in Ohio, suggesting that such constructions would eventually lead to an emergency situation.

Stasis VI: Landowner Property Risk

Across each of the states' regulatory risk reporting tools, participants noted that there is very little deliberative capacity for property owners. For example, property owners were concerned about their property rights in regard to HVHF. Some public participants, specifically property owners, wanted to know where they might find information about protecting those rights through a ban. Others wanted to know if there was a possibility of baseline testing to protect against HVHF risks that might emerge in the future. A stasis analysis shows that HVHF risks (a definitional "is" concern) associated with property rights are largely determined by the state decision to allow HVHF or not (a policy "ought" concern).

Pennsylvania

Diane, a Pennsylvania participant, found that she and her husband would have to sell their family farm due to surrounding HVHF activity. In particular, Diane discussed the pooling rules, which were readily found on Pennsylvania's institutional sites, that would force HVHF activity under her farm through horizontal drilling techniques: "And then when we were going through all of that with forced pooling, they were literally sending edicts down by the hour . . . and they are all on this page . . . on this gas pooling page." Here, HVHF risk due to horizontal fracking was not acknowledged (an "is" concern), leading to policies that forced HVHF activity under her farm (an "ought" concern).

By contrast, a participant from New York, Sally, reported that she had contemplated selling her home because of possible HVHF activity but changed her mind after New York banned HVHF drilling (an "ought" concern) based on HVHF risk (an "is" concern). Here, the choices of a homeowner were drastically different. Several were concerned about possible lower property values due to HVHF. Despite the lack of property risk representation, there is ample evidence of permitting for industry *on* individual properties—and the attendant economic rights of a landowner who would like to frack. But there was little guidance for other actors whose identities might orient them to values that lead them to reject HVHF on their property. There was no information about the rights of renters, for example. Also, all participants noted the right to a positive relationship with their natural environment. Participants were frustrated that there was little to no representation beyond what landowners could do after permitting in terms of potential HVHF light, sound, air, and water, and so on. pollution. In other words, HVHF activity was assumed for areas adjacent to, and at times even on or under a landowner's land. Diane had no control over pipelines built under her property: "Pipelines, oh these pipelines . . . they're crossing wetlands and environmentally sensitive streams . . . that noxious crap that's running through these pipelines in front of my house."

Within environmental risk participatory mechanisms, landowners could pursue regulation to moderate HVHF activity after HVHF proceeded, but most "regulations" related to property could be tempered with a variance, as Diane from Pennsylvania revealed:

> You know how they [DEP] tell that there are all these rules and regs . . . they have to be 300 ft. from your house and all this. I've never seen any rule or reg that they couldn't issue a variance against. If they (landowners) want to . . . all they have to do is apply for it. They get all these variances or releases that say, sure, you can go ahead and put that 150 ft. from their house.

Diane noted that this was a concern when property owners allowed permit variances that might affect a neighboring property. Property owners like Diane found they could not ban local HVHF that might affect personal property once drilling was given a green light in a particular state: "They don't tell you about it [banning HVHF] here [DEP site]. Oh no, that's like the underground. No, they don't say, 'Oh, if you don't like this just go ahead and object.' Oh no."

Property owners' agency in representing risks that might impact their land depended upon definitions of risk ("is") that led to state regulations about

HVHF ("ought"). Ohio and Pennsylvania property owners generally did not have agency to determine HVHF risks on personal property. While some Pennsylvania residents are currently in court over alleged water contamination on private property by an industry, it is up to the resident to prove the risk, not the industry (see table 2.2).

Additionally, I explored the stasis of human health, which will be explored more clearly in chapter 3.

SIGNIFICANCE OF INSTITUTIONAL ENVIRONMENTAL AUTHORITY BASED ON STASIS ANALYSIS

As noted before and what is clear through the stasis analysis above, authority to represent and regulate HVHF risk does not lie with local governments or, often, even federal entities. Instead, HVHF is largely defined, valued, and regulated by state agencies who, particularly in Pennsylvania and Ohio, tout the ability to regulate HVHF activity. Fischer (2000) refers to Wimer (1977) to critique the way in which one might "conflate technological advance with social progress" (p. 13). The same might be true of state institutional approaches to HVHF technology. State regulatory bodies are generally the authority in establishing risk (there are a few communities with "charters" that do regulate local risks) and state institutions regularly refer to positivist notions of obtaining knowledge: "social problems, conceptualized in technical terms, are freed from the cultural, psychological, and linguistic contexts that constitute the social tradition" via abstract language (p. 17). Participants, however, complained that science was used selectively by these states, with regulatory bodies citing studies to support or enable industrial systems vs. critique systems for the health of the environment or people. Similarly, participants noted the lack of baseline studies or cumulative studies of risks through time. This became abundantly clear when health experts in the state of New York found HVHF drilling production to pose various risks, which resulted in the state ban, but such policies were not adopted in Ohio or Pennsylvania. As such, Fischer (2000) cautions the assumption that positivist science is gone: "Basic to neopositivism and its rationalistic worldview has been an ambitious (if not arrogant) epistemological assumption: that the positivist method is the *only* valid means of obtaining 'true knowledge'" (p. 17).

Fischer calls the assumptions about neopositivism "an illusion of cultural and historical transcendence" (p. 17), which I believe plays out in this data in terms of the positivist approach to risk in all states I study that, as participants note, do not take into account complex systems that threaten neat models of environmental "management" within HVHF. For example, data sets used by experts to create HVHF policy might compartmentalize risk (risks to air might be separated from risks to water), showing only "parts" of risk factors that fail to tell a cumulative story of risk. Similarly, only certain "kinds" of scientific inquiry and risk, usually those that are friendly to the industry, are the dominant "ethos" in terms of what is represented on institutional sites. According to activists, science found on institutional sites is limited to a pro-"industry" science versus varied science experts theorizing different types of risk or intersectional risks. While many activists found local universities to be of some help in exploring questions of fact, there was considerable concern by all activists that some scientists or parts of science programs were more interested in promoting an industry vs. critically investigating an industry to explore risk—even risks local landowners were experiencing. Simmons argues that the federal EPA process is largely a one-way model of communication: "The agency's model implies a one-way flow of technical information that positions members of the public as consumers and entities to be managed" (2007, p. 13). Simmons continues by referring to "technocratic" models of risk communication by which technical experts make decisions that result in a particular environmental policy or decision (2007). This technocratic approach is seen throughout the HVHF policy process in all three states. Yet, Simmons references Winner, who sees the ambiguity among experts themselves, and questions ideological alignments: "Different fields of research give very different estimates of possible hazards" and "expertise is linked to and biased by particular social interests" (2007, p. 75). Simmons discusses the limitations of "expertise" in that ". . . experts are often defined in the most limited sense," noting that "even scientists and engineers who work in unrelated areas" tend to disagree about policy (2007, p. 88). While Simmons suggests that top-down models faded the 1980s, my research shows that reliance on fuzzy notions of expertise is still very much a force in 2017.

The authority of science to dictate risk policy becomes ambiguous depending upon who is using science and for what purpose. As the New York health stasis analysis reveals, public health science claims might contrast with geologic science claims, resulting in differing policies depending on how environmental institutions orient science claims. Similarly, in my study, science efforts by local citizens (citizen science) in conjunction with academic studies about HVHF risk shared by participants in public settings were often not recognized, and according to some participants, were attacked. Participants were often told they don't "understand science" or were voicing "opinions" vs. "facts." But participants countered that regulatory institutions "cherry-picked" certain types of science procedures that privileged a gas infrastructure vs. pursuing possibilities for alternative energy infrastructure. The result was an uncritical embrace of oil and gas development with little acknowledgment of the volatility of economics or environmental processes. Similarly, participants were often experts themselves, not an uneducated public. Simmons, instead, suggests that "the public itself must be seen as complicated, diverse, and multifaceted because a homogeneous notion of the public fails to acknowledge vastly different perspectives different members bring to a particular debate" (2007, p. 87). Acknowledgment of a more multifaceted public might reveal the potential of community groups of informed citizens, who are positioned to have expertise in local ecologies. Young (1990) notes that such expertise among citizens is possible through intersecting scholarship inquiry, "Community groups challenging the decision to construct a hazardous waste disposal site must acquire considerable technical knowledge of waste management, local geology, and law in order to conduct their campaign; in the process they discover that these matters can be understood by ordinary citizens, and that experts are rarely neutral" (p. 84).

My stasis analysis, as informed by participant commentary, reveals the overwhelming consensus from participants using Ohio and Pennsylvania state institutional sites is that institutions representing the HVHF industry position it as a "safe" activity, regulated by the environmental institutions in each state. But policies rely heavily on understudied intersecting risk concerns. New York State, in banning HVHF drilling, acknowledges that intersecting risk concerns do pose risks to human health. This comparison to states that do not make such risk claims, as displayed through patterns found in primary data, highlights the socially situated nature of HVHF risk construction within public deliberation and questions institutional mechanisms that create policy based on institutional authority.

APPENDIX: TABLES

CDA Coding

Discourse analysis is key for understanding issues of power surrounding Wodak and Meyer (2009) refer to Glaser and Strauss's (1967) notion of Grounded Theory to encourage reexamination of data as patterns emerge. This book is informed by notions of Grounded Theory, so while I entered into CDA analysis with a plan to seek patterns of normalizing discourse patterns that explicitly or implicitly create consent to neoliberal ideology frames of environmental policy through legitimation of neoliberalism, I reexamined patterns as they emerged from participant discussion, participant analysis of a text or procedure, or my own analysis of a text or procedure that a participant referred to.

Table 2.2 Stasis

Stasis I: Chemical risks

Question of . . .	OHIO	PA	New York
Fact **Are there chemical risks related to HVHF.?**	Yes, as noted in fluid disclosure documents	Possibly, chemicals must be listed on FracFocus disclosure site	Yes, as noted in the moratorium at the time of study
Definition **What are the chemical risks?**	Unclear, not represented	While some chemicals are disclosed voluntarily, should companies claim trade secrets, disclosure is not require	At time of study, under review
Value **Should there be action based on chemical risks?**	No "plan" for emergency workers to access the ways in which chemicals might interact. According to activists, very burdensome.	According to PA state Act 13, medical professionals must sign a non-disclosure form in order to see chemicals (to protect trade secrets)	At time of study, under review
Jurisdiction **What is the action suggested based on what authority?**	HVHF regulation via ODNR	HVHF regulation via PA DEP	DEC bans HVHF in the state of New York

Stasis II: Contamination risks—water and soil

Question of . . .	Ohio	PA	New York
Fact **Are there contamination risks—water, soil, or otherwise-- related to HVHF. waste?**	Ohio EPA does not consider fracking as part of its water protection plan unless the activity might impact a waterway; Data requests for HVHF are not considered a part of the Ohio EPA. Even if activity might impact air or water, the Ohio EPA generally "authorizes" or permits that activity.	Yes, as noted in legislation in 2011 banning fracking waste from wastewater treatment plants	At time of study, under review
Definition **What are the contamination risks?**	These wastes are defined as "contaminated soils" vs. "hazardous waste" by the ODNR—meaning these wastes can be disposed of in solid waste facilities.	The wastes are defined via federal EPA and applied to 2011 legislation, which notes there can be contaminants that are radioactive and might harm humans health	At time of study, under review

Value **Should there be action based on contamination risks?**	Regulation through ODNR	Regulation through PA DEP	At time of study, under review
Jurisdiction **What actions will take place based on contamination risks based on what authority?**	Disposal is permitted at solid waste facilities Some reused (recycled) via ODNR permitting	Disposal is permitted at solid waste facilities under solid waste disposal requirements Some reused (recycled) via PA DEP permitting	HVHF banned, some disposal allowed in the state of NY, regulation through NY DEC

Stasis III: Radioactivity

Questions of	OH	PA	NY
Fact **Are there radioactivity risks in HVHF production or disposal?**	Yes, but risks are minimized (Issues with the ways in which NORM (naturally occurring radioactive material) and TENORM (technically enhanced radioactive material) are defined, tested, and regulated)	Yes, but discussion of risks are minimized	Yes, but risks are minimized "New York excludes NORM from regulations requiring specialized disposal and discharge of radioactive material, unless it is 'processed and concentrated." (Steinzor and Baizel, 2015, p. 116). As a result, state laws governing the disposal of low-level radioactive waste do not apply to drill cuttings.
Definition **What are the radioactivity risks?**	Ohio's TENORM testing is uneven, specifically in regard to "earthen material" resulting from the drilling process or to brine (Steinzor and Baizel, 2015, p. 119-120); the state's legal definition of drill cuttings acknowledges that they "may include a minimum amount of fluid that results from a drilling process" (Steinzor and Baizel, 2015, p. 121)	DEP does consider TENORM to be a risk if disposal is improper (Steinzor and Baizel, 2015, p. 22), but outsources much disposal to Ohio	None articulated, but does not widely accept disposal waste.

(*Continued*)

Table 2.2 Continued

Value **Should possible radioactive risks be considered in terms of policy?**	"Regulatory agencies in Ohio prohibit operators from disposing of TENORM waste at well sites, and disposal facilities can only accept wastes that have concentrations at less than 5 pCi/g above background levels—although this requirement does not apply to wastes that ODNR defines as NORM." (Steinzor and Baizel, 2015, p. 117)	None articulated, but does not widely accept HVHF waste disposal	None articulated, but does not widely accept HVHF waste disposal.
Jurisdiction **What actions about radioactivity will take place based on what authority?**	Ohio's regulatory agencies have done little testing of oil and gas field wastes to determine their radioactivity content, particularly with regard to the Utica Shale. Regulation through ODNR	None articulated, Regulation through PA DEP	Some waste accepted. Regulation through NY DEC

Stasis IV: Seismic activity risk

Question of . . .	**OH**	**PA**	**NY**
Fact **Are there seismic risks related to HVHF.?**	"Following a series of over 100 earthquakes in northeastern Ohio in 2011-2012—12 of which registered at nearly 2 and one almost 4 on the Richter scale—researchers at Columbia University confirmed the cause to be drilling wastewater disposal at a large injection well." (Steinzor and Baizel, 2015, p. 33) Though studies by the ODNR itself make a direct case between earthquakes and injection wells, this is not clearly reflected on the ODNR page	Yes	Under review at the time of study
Definition **What are the seismic risks?**	The risks are framed as minimal	Minor	Under review at the time of study

Value **Should there be actions based on seismic risks?**	in 2012, ODNR and legislators revised the Ohio Administrative Code to require operators of deep underground injection wells in certain formations (ranging from about 1,000–13,000 feet) to survey the location for potential faults, submit a plan for monitoring seismic activity, conduct pressure tests, and potentially limit the rate and volume of injection Stronger permitting, but continue activity (see table 2.2 Continued)	"EPA has recently issued several permits for UIC wells in the state, with others likely to follow; in doing so, the agency has indicated that the wells would be unlikely to cause seismic activity due to the pumping pressure and well depth that operators included in their permit applications." (Steinzor and Baizel, 2015, p. 34).	NY DEC
Jurisdiction **What actions will proceed based on what authority?**	Suspend, but do not ban activities as regulated through ODNR	Continue activity with oversight, as regulated through PA DEP	Continue limited activity, as regulated through NY DEC

Stasis V: Injection well risks

	OH	PA	NY
Fact **Are there injection well risks related to HVHF?**	Yes –	Yes –	Under review at the time of study
Definition **What are the injection well risks?**	The risks are framed as minimal—earthquake, soil, and water	The risks are framed as minimal—earthquake, soil, and water	Under review at the time of study
Value **Should there be action based on injection well risks?**	State regulation	State regulation	State regulation
Jurisdiction **What actions will proceed based on what authority?**	If problematic, suspend but do not ban activities as regulated through ODNR	Continue activity with oversight, as regulated through DEP	Continue limited activity, as regulated through NY DEC

(Continued)

Table 2.2 Continued

Stasis VI: Landowner property risk

Questions of:	**OH**	**PA**	**NY**
Fact **Are there landowner property value risks?**	No representation on ODNR site	No representation on PA DEP site	No representation on NY DEC site
Definition **What are the property value risks?**	See above	See above	See above
Value **Should there be action based on property risks?**	No statewide plan (baseline testing, etc.)	No statewide plan (baseline testing, etc.)	See above
Jurisdiction **What is the action suggested based on what authority?**	See above ODNR regulates HVHF	PA DEP regulates HVHF; Dimock, PA residents move to federal EPA and . . . .Hazardous materials lawsuits against the company (water on private property)	NY DEC bans HVHF in the state of New York

Table 2.3 Rationale for Analytical Categories

Participant Concern	*Reporting Number*	*Analytical Category*
Participant concern about institutional authority and regulation as seen through permitting *for* HVHF	Reported by eighteen participants	Discourse legitimation through "expert authority" and "impersonal authority"
Participant concern about the way in which HVHF activity is normalized as seen through permitting *for* HVHF	Reported by eighteen participants	Discourse legitimation through "explanation"
Participant concern about institutional authority and regulation in terms of complex HVHF risk and positioning of nature as subordinate to human problem solving	Reported by eighteen participants	Administrative rationalism discourse (metaphors and erasures)
Participant concern about how HVHF is largely valued through the capitalist economic system	Reported by thirteen participants	Economic rationalism discourse (metaphors and erasures)
Participant identification of precautionary discourse within HVHF deliberation	Reported by five participants (all from NY)	Green politics discourse (comparative example)

As noted in table 2.3, one notable pattern that emerged early on as defined by all eighteen participants was that of the ways in which institutions are positioned to grant permitting *for* various aspects of HVHF activity versus banning portions of an uncertain HVHF activity. In this case, I pay close attention to patterns in the language of texts and processes participants navigate that might "legitimate" power, specifically the power to permit *for* HVHF industry activity because of an assumed shared value: such as monetary gain from the activity. State institutional sites often legitimize the "permitting" of selected unconventional gas activities (van Dijk, 2003, p. 360). Similarly, I also found a pattern within the way discourse structures were positioned to "guide" participants to "normalized" (as defined by institutions) interactions (van Dijk, 2003, p. 358) based on this legitimation. To code for discursive legitimation patterns as grounded in a neoliberal orientation found through participant interviews and TAPs, I turn to van Leeuwen's (2007) legitimation framework, notably patterns of "authoritization" legitimation and "rationalization" legitimation (p. 91).

By investigating patterns of "authorization" legitimation, the content of interviews and TAPs led me to code for ways by which legitimation of HVHF occurs in environmental risk participatory mechanisms through "expert legitimation." Here, I coded for discursive expert positioning as a rationale for HVHF activity by looking for patterns of, as van Leeuwen notes, the position of expert in a text, "Typically, expert legitimation takes the form of 'verbal process clauses' or 'mental process clauses' (e.g., 'Professor so-and-so believes. . .') with the expert as subject." (2007, p. 95). Patterns in interviews and TAPs also led me to code for van Leeuwen's notion of "impersonal authority" by which "laws, rules, and regulations" and "policies, the guidelines" guide an outcome. Here, I coded for van Leeuwen's suggestions of patterns of language constructions that legitimize, in this case, HVHF activity:

> Impersonal authorities can be the subject of "verbal process clauses" just as readily as personal authorities ("The rules state that . . . "; "The law says that . . . "). But the indispensable element in legitimations of this kind is the presence of nouns such as "policy," "regulation," "rule," "law," etc. or their cognate adjectives and adverbs (e.g. "compulsory," "mandatory," "obligatory"), which often appear in impersonal clauses. (2007, p. 96)

All participants felt that rationalizations *for* HVHF were often subtle and presupposed HVHF industrial activity *would* occur prior to the opportunity for meaningful public deliberation. HVHF would proceed as a naturalized activity for which permits would be provided (participants noted that value systems upholding this naturalized approach are based in a neoliberal orientation toward resource extraction). This led me to code within van Leeuwen's framework of theoretical rationalization that accounts for activities framed as "the way things are" with "explicit representation" of a given activity (2007, p. 103). Within van Leeuwen's theoretical constructs, his notion of *explanation* as theoretical rationalization most closely fits patterns I observed across interviews and TAPs, that of permitting *for* HVHF activity. Thus, I chose discursive patterns of *explanation* as a coding scheme. Here, van Leeuwen highlights ways explanation works to legitimate a given position:

> Here the answer to the "why" question is, "because doing things this way is appropriate to the nature of these actors." Generality is again essential. Explanations describe general attributes or habitual activities of the categories of actors in question.

In the case of my data, this notion of "explanation" is linked to the earlier notion of legitimation through authority. In this case, actors are the institutions that claim "regulatory" expertise in HVHF activity for economic gain and discuss permitting *for* HVHF activity (which, as participants note, is a complex practice within complex systems and is rife with uncertainty). Table 2.4 outlines my discourse legitimation coding scheme.

I also approached my CDA coding by seeking ideological patterns found within discourses in the texts (official or unofficial) created by or used by public participants as they negotiate environmental risks (Cox, 2006; Dryzek, 2005, pp. 13–17). I did so because all eighteen participants voiced concern

Table 2.4 Discourse Legitimation Coding Scheme

Discourse legitimation *(van Leeuwen, 2007)*
authorization legitimation
expert legitimation:

> *"Typically, expert legitimation takes the form of 'verbal process clauses' or 'mental process clauses' (e.g., 'Professor so-and-so believes. . .') with the expert as subject." (van Leeuwen, 2007, p. 95).*

impersonal authority:

> *Impersonal authorities can be the subject of "verbal process clauses" just as readily as personal authorities ("The rules state that . . ."; "The law says that . . ."). But the indispensable element in legitimations of this kind is the presence of nouns such as "policy," "regulation," "rule," "law," etc. or their cognate adjectives and adverbs (e.g. "compulsory," "mandatory," "obligatory"), which often appear in impersonal clauses. (van Leeuwen, 2007, p. 96).*

Combined, institutions in this study are presented as impersonal expert authorities (see underlined portion in the example below)

Ex: *ODNR-DOGRM regulates brine disposal in Ohio.*

rationalization legitimation, theoretical legitimation
explanation:

> *"Here the answer to the 'why' question is, 'because doing things this way is appropriate to the nature of these actors'. Generality is again essential. Explanations describe general attributes or habitual activities of the categories of actors in question." (van Leeuwen, 2007, p. 104)*

(See underlined portion in the example below)

Ex: *The Ohio Department of Natural Resources, Division of Oil and Gas Resource Management (ODNR-DOGRM) has primary regulatory authority over oil and gas drilling activity in Ohio, including rules for well construction, design and operation.*

about value systems within environmental risk participatory mechanisms that were at odds with their own, particularly in terms of what participants felt to be the lack of value on human and ecological health within institutional risk participatory mechanisms. Within these discourses, I coded for Dryzek's construction of "storylines," or ontologies, assumptions, and agents and their motives related to "ideological patterns that revealed particular ideologies through linguistic choices" (Dryzek, 2005, pp. 17–18). Similarly, I look at Dryzek's notion of "assumptions about natural relationships" by which "discourses embody notions of what is natural in the relationships between different entities. Some see competition, be it between human beings in markets or between creatures locked in Darwinian struggle, as natural. Others see cooperation as the essence of both human social systems and natural systems" (2005, p. 18). Finally, I adopt Dryzek's construct of analyzing environmental "agents and their motives." According to Dryzek, "Storylines require actors, or agents. These actors can be individuals or collectives. They are mostly human, but can be nonhuman" (2005, p. 18).

For example, does a particular risk reporting site or procedure reveal an ideology through discourse in which humans are able to dominate "matter" which is regulated through technology and markets? (Promethean view) (Dryzek, 2005, p. 60–61). Do risk reporting sites and procedures yield language patterns that reveal other ideologies about the way in which humans position themselves within, or, at times, outside of "the environment": administrative rationalism, democratic pragmatism, economic rationalism, sustainability, ecological modernization, or even green radicalism (Dryzek, 2005)? By using discourse analysis, I found evidence of relationships between humans and "nature" or "the environment" as defined and positioned by various institutional risk reporting tools and procedures that legitimized particular policies within institutional participatory tools.

To code for this study, I adopted a theoretical framework and coded for two environmental discourse storylines in particular that fit many participants' concerns about environmental risk participatory mechanisms as revealed through the retrospective interviews and the TAP: Dryzek's (2005) administrative rationalism and economic rationalism (see table 2.4). These schemes reveal how participants struggled to find value systems within environmental risk mechanisms that might enact policies informed by precaution or environmental justice. To showcase the comparative nature of competing discourses among states, I also analyzed a rare document found among risk participatory mechanisms that highlights environmental justice considerations by using Dryzek's (2005) green politics storyline (see table 2.4). Only one TAP from New York revealed a document using this scheme, but all five participants from New York discussed the way in which public health concerns were central in banning HHVHF.

Additionally, extending these storylines, I analyze using the notion of what Arran Stibbe refers to as "metaphors" and "erasures." Both Arran Stibbe (2016) and John Dryzek (2005) describe metaphors as comparisons through language that create "frames" for thought and eventual action. Of central importance is what is being compared in terms of "source" and "target" domains (Stibbe, 2016). In other words, metaphors can evoke powerful ways of thinking about certain natural phenomena. Stibbe calls attention to different ways climate change (the target) can be framed within source domains: as violence against plant, animal, and human species, as a greenhouse occurrence, and as a roller coaster among many (2016, pp. 65–66). The way the metaphorical frames are constructed, linguistically, links to how the general public uses logic.

Erasures, according to Stibbe (2015), are language constructions that create a mindset that "an area of life is unimportant or untrustworthy" (p. 202). In particular, Stibbe points to the systemic "erasure" of natural phenomenon within discourse, making certain ideas seem "marginal" or "unimportant" (p. 145–146). When discourses about economics only champion material costs versus a rich description and valuing of the natural world, there is an erasure. I fold both metaphors and erasures into categories created by Dryzek (2005): Basic entities, assumptions about natural relationships, and agents and their motives (see table 2.5).

Table 2.5 Administrative Rationalism Discourse Coding Scheme and Economic Rationalism Coding Scheme

Administrative Rationalism *(Dryzek, 2005, p. 89)*
I. Basic entities recognized or constructed (informing ideology)
Liberal capitalism
Administrative state
Experts
Managers (see underlined portion in the example below)
II. Assumptions about natural relationships
Nature subordinate to human problem solving
People subordinate to state
Experts and managers control state (see italicized *portion in the example below)*
III. Agents and their motives
Experts and managers

Ex: *The Ohio Department of Natural Resources, Division of Oil and Gas Resource Management (ODNR-DOGRM)* has primary regulatory authority over oil and gas drilling activity in Ohio, *including rules for well construction, design and operation.*
Metaphors: *Nature is subordinate to human problem solving (ODNR)*
Erasures: *Nature has no agency, is not considered*

Economic Rationalism *(Dryzek, 2005, p. 133)*

I. Basic entities recognized or constructed (informing ideology)
Homo economicus [1] *(see underlined portion in the example below)*
Markets
Prices
Property
Governments (not citizens)
II. Assumptions about natural relationships
Competition
Hierarchy based on expertise (see italicized *portion in the example below)*
Subordination of nature
III. Agents and their motives
Homo economicus: self interested
Some government officials must be motivated by the public interest
Ex: *If a company is interested in beneficially reusing contaminated soils,* it must get authorization for this activity from Ohio EPA's Division of Materials and Waste Management (DMWM) . . .
Metaphors: *Nature is subordinate to economic issues (beneficial reuse of soils in the company interest)*
Erasures: *Soil (nature) is acted upon vs. having innate value*

(Continued)

Table 2.5 (Continued)

By contrast, Green Politics *(Dryzek, 2005, p. 218)*

I. Basic entities recognized or constructed (informing ideology)
Global limits
Nature as complex ecosystems
Humans with broad capacities
Social, economic, and political structures
II. Assumptions about natural relationships
Equality among people
Complex interconnections between humans and nature (see underlined *portion in the example below)*
Subordination of nature
/II. Agents and their motives
Many individual and collective actors, multidimensional motivation (see italicized *portion in the example below)*
Agency in nature downplayed though not necessarily denied.

Ex*: In this instance, however, the overall weight of the evidence from the* cumulative body of information contained in this Public Health Review *demonstrates that there are significant uncertainties about the kinds of adverse health outcomes that may be associated with HVHF . . .*
Metaphors*: Communication about nature is complex and emerging within several social structures*

[1] According to Dryzek, Homo economicus highlights a belief in a world "populated by economic actors" who might "appear as a consumer or a producer; and if the producers are organized into firms, the firm still behaves like an individual" (p. 133). In this ideology, markets are preferable to politics. Similarly, material and personal benefits are highlighted.

In coding for legitimation and administrative rationalism, economic rationalism or green politics discourses, I situate my analysis in Wodak and Meyer's notion that "CDA frequently detects the linguistic means used by the privileged to stabilize or even to intensify inequities in society. This entails careful systematic analysis, and self-reflection at every point of one's research and distance from the data which are being investigated" (2009, p. 32). As such, I analyze the TAP screenshots in use, allowing participants to guide analysis given participant critiques of environmental risk participatory mechanisms captured by TAP and informed by retrospective interviews.

As with rhetorical analysis, as I work through my CDA analysis, I provided examples from public participant interviews or TAPs to showcase rhetorical patterns that emerge from the "no" and the "yes" responses in terms of limitations to deliberation within environmental participatory mechanisms. When applicable, I included commentary from participants themselves about issues of legitimation and discourse storylines and patterns of metaphors and erasures. However, I also further analyzed texts participants might have led me to, as participants were not discourse scholars and our interviews and TAPs were not designed for participants to perform discourse analysis. It is from this participant-sourced data that I chose to conduct further analysis. I include a sample CDA analysis as revealed in a screenshot from Peg's TAP below (see table 2.6).

Table 2.6 CDA Analysis

CDA Analysis
1. *What patterns of power are revealed within the reporting tools?*
a. discourse legitimation (van Leeuwen, 2007)
-authorization (expert authority; impersonal authority)
-rationalization (explanation)
b. discourse storylines: (Dryzek, 2005) - Administrative rationalism - Economic rationalism - Comparative case (rare): green politics
Metaphors and erasures:
-basic entities informing an ideology
- assumptions about natural relationships
- agents and their motive

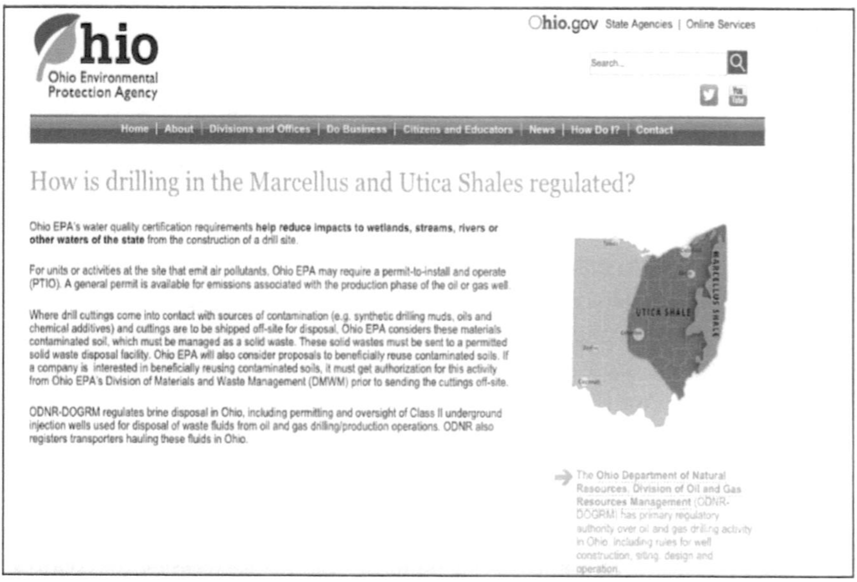

Figure 2.2 Representative Sample, Peg's TAP. *Source*: Screenshot by author

For the analysis below, I use a representative sample from a think-aloud protocol with a participant named Peg who reviewed the ODNR page, which I include as a screenshot below (figure 2.2).

Legitimation

Peg read the following text from the ODNR website:

> Where drill cuttings come into contact with sources of contamination (e.g. synthetic drilling muds, oils and chemical additives) and cuttings are to be shipped off-site for disposal, *Ohio EPA* considers these materials contaminated soil,

> which must be managed as a solid waste. These solid wastes must be sent to a permitted solid waste disposal facility. *Ohio EPA* will also *consider proposals* to beneficially reuse contaminated soils. If a company is interested in beneficially reusing contaminated soils, it must get *authorization* for this activity from *Ohio EPA's Division of Materials and Waste Management (DMWM)* prior to sending the cuttings off-site.
>
> *ODNR-DOGRM regulates* brine disposal in Ohio, including *permitting and oversight of Class II underground injection wells* used for disposal of waste fluids from oil and gas drilling/production operations. *ODNR* also *registers* transporters hauling these fluids in Ohio.
>
> *The Ohio Department of Natural Resources, Division of Oil and Gas Resource Management (ODNR-DOGRM)* has *primary regulatory authority over oil and gas drilling activity in Ohio,* including *rules* for well construction, design and operation.

Above, I show Peg's interaction with the screenshot shared in figure 2.2. Peg responds to the italicized portions of the text she is reading. Here, Peg expresses frustration in terms of which agency she might report HVHF risks to. While the Ohio EPA deals with environmental protection, Peg reiterates that this does not ultimately extend to HVHF activity; rather, the Ohio Department of Natural Resources has the final say in HVHF regulation: "The ODNR has primacy." When Peg attempts to link to the ODNR from this OH EPA site, she discusses the ways in which state environmental institutions send users between sites, resulting in confusion and frustration for public participants attempting to use sites, "They always do, it's like a big hamster wheel . . . ODNR, ODNR . . . Go to ODNR because we [OH EPA] don't [regulate] risks."

Here, I analyze the way in which state institutions legitimize themselves by positioning themselves as expert authorities that can regulate HVHF. Either the Ohio EPA or the Ohio Department of Natural Resources is repeated as subjects in each sentence: "Ohio EPA," a division of the Ohio EPA called the "DMWM," or the "The Ohio Department of Natural Resources, Division of Oil and Gas Resource Management." Additionally, while the state agencies are named, they are impersonal—no names are given of who might design or implement these complex regulations. Here, I also analyze the ways in which legitimation occurs by the state agencies' use of impersonal authorities by noting the verbal clauses following the unnamed expert subject. Regulatory actions are carried out by unnamed state experts, as noted by the underlined phrases: "manage[d]," "consider proposals" gives "authorization," "regulates," allows for "permitting and oversight," "registers," "has primary regulatory authority," and establishes "rules." These actions suggest regulation by an expert agency, the authority, though there is considerable confusion by public participants about how these regulations came to be, why certain state agencies have power over others, and why regulations overwhelmingly position HVHF as an assumed activity.

Additionally, Peg read the following ODNR text:

> ODNR-DOGRM regulates brine disposal in Ohio, including permitting and oversight of *Class II underground injection wells used for disposal of waste fluids from oil and gas drilling/production operations.* ODNR also registers *transporters hauling these fluids in Ohio.* The Ohio Department of Natural Resources, Division of Oil and Gas Resource Management (ODNR-DOGRM) has primary_regulatory authority over oil and gas drilling activity in Ohio, including rules for *well construction, design and operation.*

Peg made the following comment:

> The ODNR has primacy. They always do, it's like a big hamster wheel . . . ODNR, ODNR . . . Go to ODNR because we [OH EPA] don't [regulate] risks.

Here, I focus more closely on the portion that Peg discussed in her TAP to understand the HVHF activities that are legitimized. One of Peg's frustrations in looking at this screenshot was the lack of discussion of precaution and risk of HVHF. HVHF activity was simply assumed with little oversight. As she read the bolded portion above, she mused, as shown in the italicized portion to the left, "we [Ohio EPA] don't [regulate] risks."

In further analysis of Peg's TAP, I turn to "explanation" legitimation to consider what activities, exactly, the authority is regulating and how this site legitimizes specific HVHF activities. Here, I find language that positions general or habitual HVHF activities as standard practice, when some of these activities are, in fact, regulated very differently (or not allowed at all) in other states. The italicized portions reference HVHF activities that are framed as habitual. The phrases "Class II underground injection wells used for disposal of waste fluids from oil and gas drilling/production operations" and "transporters hauling these fluids in Ohio" both refer to injection wells; public participants in Ohio argue that Ohio bears a disproportionate share of accepting HVHF fluid waste in injection wells as compared to neighboring states, so this activity is questioned as being normalized. Similarly, the text Peg read above refers to "well construction, design and operation" as a standard activity that occurs in Ohio, when HVHF wells are illegal in New York. Thus, "explanation" legitimation positions HVHF activity as habitual action when it is, in fact, highly contested. Patterns of legitimation found in this study overwhelmingly greenlit permitting,

As mentioned earlier in this chapter, Peg was frustrated because she did not know which institutional agency she might report HVHF risks to. While the Ohio EPA deals with environmental protection, Peg reiterates that this does not ultimately extend to HVHF activity; rather, the Ohio Department of Natural Resources has the final say in HVHF regulation, leading to Peg's comment, "The ODNR has primacy" (italicized). As she read the bold portions above, Peg's recognition of the hierarchies within state institutions lends itself to an analysis of administrative rationalism discourse found in the text.

In my analysis, I refer to underlined portions of the text above to reveal administrative rationalism discourse that encourages HVHF activity, a discourse that pervades all institutional sites represented in this study. Here, the metaphor is that of the institution as having control of nature. Here, actors are managers and experts, and nature is erased in terms of having any kind of agency or value beyond a commodity: instead, it is seen as something to be "managed." In the excerpt above, agents and their motives are experts and managers, such as the "Ohio EPA" or the "ODNR." These experts or managers assume that nature is subordinate to human problem-solving. "Contaminated soils" are "managed as a solid waste" in a "solid waste disposal facility," which assumes that soils might remain static in a facility, an assumption about which many public participants were highly suspicious. Another instance of the subordination of nature to human problem-solving appears in the discussion of underground injection wells. Here, the expert ODNR "regulates" brine disposal by "permitting" *for* "underground injection wells," which are used "for disposal of waste fluids from oil and gas drilling/production operations." Here, there are implicit assumptions that underground injection wells are safe, and that fluids will remain static in the wells. This assumption was a concern for many participants. Finally, I look at how administrative rationalism discourse positions experts and managers that control the state. The statement "Ohio Department of Natural Resources, Division of Oil and Gas Resource Management (ODNR-DOGRM) has primary regulatory authority over oil and gas drilling activity in Ohio" explicitly denies the Ohio EPA (which has established water, soil, and air standards) authority over oil and gas drilling. This position is very troubling to participants like Peg who come to the Ohio EPA page to learn about possible protections, only to learn that the language is oriented *toward* HVHF activity.

Economic Rationalism Discourse Patterns—Metaphors/Erasures

Peg also read the following lines from the ODNR website:

> Ohio's EPA water quality certification requirements help reduce impacts to wetlands, streams, rivers, or other waters of the state from the construction of a drill site . . . . Ohio EPA will also consider proposals to beneficially reuse contaminated soils. If a company is interested in beneficially reusing contaminated soils, it must get authorization for this activity from Ohio EPA's Division of Materials and Waste Management (DMWM) prior to sending the cuttings off-site.

I focus on this excerpt, which Peg read but did not comment on, to showcase language constructs that reveal economic rationalism discourse. My analysis of the text above indicates economic rationalism discourse. Here, the metaphor is clear in terms of the Ohio EPA as an entity that is comprised of markets and properties. Nature is subordinated to the interests of market prices. The concept of the value of nature is entirely erased in this scenario.

The OH EPA never considers *not* drilling as an option to proceed with HVHF activity. Instead, the EPA represents a government agency motivated by the public interest of "helping to reduce impacts" but not *stop* impacts of "from the construction of a drill site." There is no language to indicate that the public interest might be to avoid drilling altogether or to consider any activity beyond the time frame of the "construction" phase of a drill site, subordinating nature such as "wetlands, streams, rivers or other waters" to the inevitable drill site. Bypassing HVHF altogether is not part of the Ohio EPA protection plan.

The selection above also shows examples of Homo economicus, which according to Dryzek, highlights a belief in a world "populated by economic actors" (2005, p. 133). Not only does the Ohio EPA not consider banning HVHF activity, it views byproducts of HVHF as a possible commodity where "companies" might "beneficially reuse contaminated soils" through "authorization" of a state institution. As little is known about the long-term effects of HVHF byproducts, such language encourages an economic system where material benefits of contaminated soils caused by HVHF activity are more clear than the "environment" itself, relying only a certification (to practice HVHF) that might only "help reduce impacts" to waterways.

Green storylines include positive and beneficial discourses and are notably absent in most examples from the interactions of participants in Ohio and PA. In chapter 3, I discuss how participants find ways to reframe risk communication to include their local concerns.

NOTES

1. Bäckstrand notes, "Risk assessment is still regarded as the exclusive domain for science experts" (2003, p. 34).

2. Schiappa outlines this is/ought construction within the discussion of rhetorical analysis of definition: "A rhetorical analysis of definition, then, investigates how people persuade other people to adopt and use certain definitions to the exclusion of others" (1998, p. 2). In this study, I focus on the is/ought portion of Schiappa's discussion of definition.

3. Schiappa points to four federal regulatory agencies with "legislative or administrative power to define wetlands according to their respective needs and interests" (2003, p. 26).

Chapter 3

Linguistic Frames

Stories from Ohio and Pennsylvania and the Difficulty of Revealing Environmental Risk

Simmons (2007) explores definitions of "risk communication" and public participation, noting that the current definitional status of risk communication comes from a small group of researchers who tend to privilege the notion of risk communicators as "technical experts" who transmit risk knowledge to a broader public. Simmons' concern is that this assumption about risk communication does not "value the knowledge citizens can contribute to policy," resulting in a public that is largely marginalized during risk deliberations (p. 41). Simmons suggests definitions of "risk communication" that might encourage "significant" citizen participation in environmental policy (p. 42). Thus, for chapters 3 and 4, I developed a coding scheme to analyze invented or alternative literacies participants found themselves engaged in, particularly those that allowed for precautionary or environmental frames that many did not find in institutional deliberation tools. Here, I combine both the rhetorical notion of "invention" and attendant literacy studies, though here I situate the discussion of rhetoric within literacy studies.

In choosing activists who explore alternative ways of making meaning about environmental risk, I also seek to understand new rhetorical patterns in deliberation and note examples of sustainable science, which is concerned with the emergence of more complex notions of science and decision-making by including extended peer communities in this decision-making (McGreavy, Silka, and Hart, 2012).

Public participants largely reject practices that are not inclusionary and seek other outlets; according to Simmons (2007), "In the reactionary model, risk assessors consider only the technical aspects of risk during the decision-making process, not the concerns and values of each local community, resulting in public outcry against a risk or policy" (p. 93). However, Stibbe critiques the ways in which participants are often positioned as though they are simply in a "deficit" model by which they can "act" when they have access to "information" about environmental risks. Instead, he suggests that inaction or action about an environmental risk involves "identity," or "the deeply held values and beliefs that relate to a sense of self" (2015, p. 105). In discussing counter-literacies, I must be clear about the pattern of my participants identifying as "activists" and why. Stibbe's literature review about "ecological identity" and "pro-environmental behavior" offers a way for me to theorize how activists made the decision to engage in counter-literacies. In the passage below, Stibbe refers to a quote by conservationist Aldo Leopold before exploring other views of ecological identity and action: "We abuse land because we regard it as a commodity. When we see land as a community to which we belong we may begin to use it with love and respect" (2015, p. 114–115).

My participants revealed personal ties to ecosystems in many ways that led them to shift to an activist identity. My interviews revealed that activists were moved to action because they held worldviews that led them to take action to protect ecological space, ecological health, and human health.

POSITIVE AND BENEFICIAL DISCOURSES IN OHIO AND PENNSYLVANIA—SALIENCE AND RE-MINDING

My study takes an interventionist turn in that I detail how public participants engage in counter-literacies in an effort to make more transparent decision-making about hydraulic fracturing and its attendant infrastructure. Public participants offer alternatives to hydraulic fracturing systems by considering alternative energy systems. My study challenges assumptions about public participation, which routinely deny citizens the opportunity to join in meaningful deliberation about environmental issues that will impact them in material ways. Sauer (2003) suggests that researchers might look more deeply at ways varied participants might communicate about "particular problems of work, risk, authority, uncertainty, and disaster" to "make visible those marginalized forms of representations that might not be visible with conventional forms of analysis" (p. 6). Similarly, Long's (2009) work with community action within rhetorics of environmentalism, community action literacies, and public engagement reveals situated, or contextualized local knowledges which are uniquely positioned to "invent" ways of making meaning about the environment that are often lost in traditional risk reporting mechanisms sponsored by local, state, or federal institutions. This is an important consideration in my study as public participants sought ways to make meaning about their local and material environments with which they had a considerable expertise. Long's discussion of how "counter-public discourse" and literacies among groups who may have been struggling to represent risk within traditional risk reporting mechanisms reveals an alternative to institutionalized discourses; these offer the opportunity for marginalized voices to offer expertise in public discourse to build a stronger articulation of risk.

In my study, I look closely at the notion of invention and these counterpublic discourses. Many scholars seek possibilities of more active participation in such discourses as informed by feminist studies:

> As a response to the marginalization felt by participants, I explore texts and procedures that participants create in their effort to "rewrite" institutional literate practice. I suggest that such texts and processes are rich places to explore in an effort to provide more inclusive processes for public participation about environmental risks, and suggest that such a feminist approach offers insights into possibilities of praxis as related to environmental risk deliberation. (George, 2017b)

Judy Wajcman's work articulating the concept of technofeminism is important in my study as it explores the social constructions questioning who might feel comfortable (or not) navigating various technical spaces and considers a feminist approach to reconsidering those spaces: "Feminist research has been at the forefront of moves to deconstruct the designer/user divide, and that between production and consumption, emphasizing the connectedness of all phases of technological development" (Cockburn and Ormrod, 1993) (Qtd. in Wajcman, 2007, p. 293).

The literacies employed by public participants navigating environmental risk are increasingly digital, technical, and networked; Herndl and Cutlip (2013) and Grabill (2007) reveal environmental activist engagement through technology that situates scientific rhetorical studies toward praxis. For this study, I look closely at this notion of aforementioned notions of "situated" and "contextualized" local literacy participants use to partake in understanding how my participants make knowledge—many of whom share literate activities online. Ultimately, I explore texts and procedures that participants create in response to the marginalization they felt by institutional reporting mechanisms in their effort to "rewrite" institutional literate practice, and suggest that such texts and processes are rich places to explore in an effort to provide more inclusive processes for public participation about environmental risks.

IN RESPONSE: ACTIVIST TECHNICAL NETWORKS

I use the term "activist technical networks" (George, 2017b) to seek insight into networks and activities participants engage in to "counter" the marginalization they feel when working with institutionalized participatory mechanisms. The activist activity often occurs in what Simmons and Grabill (2007) refer to as "distributive activities" (p. 436). Here, individuals within groups gather, then represent complex technical information to networked community groups that are "connected to larger rhetorical situations and communication practices" (Simmons and Grabill, p. 437). Research in literate practices of environmental risk reveals publics as active participants in building technological networks accessing and responding to highly technical knowledge vs. passive recipients of technical knowledge from experts. Herndl and Cutlip (2013) discuss engagement in such practices in terms of technology and the environment in situating scientific rhetorical studies toward praxis: "As Fiorino argued in 1990, including citizens in technology development and decision-making creates better technology, increases public adoption of new technologies, and supports basic democratic principles against a technocratic model of science and technology" (p. 6). Most activists in my study attended various local, and sometimes state, national, or even international events as concerned citizens, but reported a fair bit of networking occurred online to inform what was verbalized in a public setting or a publically shared text. In this collection, Oullette discusses possibilities of digital circulation, invention, and social action:

> Moving beyond the notion that rhetorics are individual speech acts, or occasion-bound events, I consider rhetoric as a larger, circulating, affective network of arguments, and thus propose that we rethink our understanding of social action on the web, and see it in terms of circulation. (2017)

Similarly, Royster and Kirsch (2012) refer to the concept of "social circulation" to situate circulation more firmly within a social context:

> we wanted a useful metaphor for re-anchoring in a more generative way the convergence of both the values added by the use of feminist ideologies in rhetoric and analyses and the use of rhetorical theories and criticism in feminist analyses, all well considered within a thickly rendered social, political economic, cultural context. (p. 23)

Additionally, Royster and Kirsch (2012) note the need for contextualizing complexities of such circulating rhetorical practices:

> Noticing . . . rather than ignoring—ecological conditions, or the ethical, political, cultural dimensions of rhetorical enterprises, or the materiality of ideas, arguments, sites, and situations, we come to *rhetoric* as an embodied polylogical social practice that needs to be understood symphonically and in high definition. (p. 94)

Understanding the ways in which alternatives to institutional risk are circulated within social constructs becomes important in terms of how activists engage in counter-literacies.

As participants sought alternatives to represent "felt" risk not represented through institutions, I began to see patterns in participants engaging in the rhetorical notion of invention, or "the ability to discover the resources for persuasion that were available in specific situation" (Cox, 2006, p. 53). In the rhetorical canon of invention, literacy heuristics or patterns aid in generating ideas about a given issue. Particular patterns of invention, as noted by Simmons and Grabill (2007), outline ways in which knowledge is built to persuade. For example, participants use particular narrative patterns to outline various arguments about the way in which humans interact with (or even within) a particular environment. Similarly, technologies such as crowd-sourced online mapping and social media allow for persuasive messages to be shared more quickly and across time and space, allowing citizens to share "models" of deliberation:

- Social Media as Technical Networks of Environmental Risk
- Multi-modality and Representation as Technical Networks of Environmental Risk
- Narratives as Networks of Environmental Risk

SOCIAL MEDIA AS TECHNICAL NETWORKS OF ENVIRONMENTAL RISK

Social media sites like Facebook were cited by many activists as a gateway for networks for other, more technical investigations. Indeed, as a community member in an area impacted by hydraulic fracturing, particularly after a seismic event, I turned to area activist group sites on Facebook to attempt to find groups that might share information that was not available on Ohio state institutional sites, including local meetings not published on state environmental sites. I also found groups that were organizing initiatives to invite the public to write letters to pressure the state to disclose earthquake data, which led to my discovering other groups pressuring the state to force companies to disclose the chemical makeup of HVHF. Many other activists sought social media to find individuals or groups who were sympathetic to similar environmental risk marginalization experiences. Others found that social media was an important space to direct activists to forums to share technical risk information revealed by academic studies not yet represented on institutional sites, and to find activists who might question, or engage in, citizen's audits, such as the audit conducted by Ohio Citizen Action which critiqued the access to meaningful risk information available on institutional sites as noted in the citizen's summary. Additionally, and also in the citizens' summary, Craig found that

> Authors of Ohio's oil and gas regulatory framework have systematically removed citizens from the process of regulating and monitoring the industry. From awarding the Ohio Department of Natural Resources (ODNR) "sole and exclusive authority" over the industry to refusing to allow public hearings on permits, Ohio's legislature has engineered a system where people don't matter. (2014, p. 3)

While there is no way to measure specific levels of "agency" through social media sites like Facebook and activist blogs or websites, these activists began to engage in groups that regularly posted updates about local, state, and federal laws; ways to gather information or critique what was represented on institutionalized sites, to find sites and processes that might represent environmental risk in more complexity than on institutionalized sites, to find emerging scientific studies about the risks about the production, storage, and transport of hydraulic fracturing materials; to understand emerging public health studies about varied risks; to investigate emerging economic studies; to find and engage in citizen science opportunities; and to find and engage with professionals (toxicologists, radiation specialists, health experts, etc.) not represented on institutionalized sites who were willing to work with concerned citizens about localized issues related to the hydraulic fracturing industry.

Tom and Bob, from Pennsylvania, who identified as educators, hunters, and fishers, worked with scientists to explore the possible long-term consequences of radioactivity in waterways of Greene County. This effort found its way into a peer-reviewed study about possible radioactive contaminants. Social media oriented activists toward spaces where they might engage in critical discussions with local higher education institutions to question the academic alignment of pro-industry research agendas, to allow activists to consider how academic institutions might engage communities in critical conversations about the uncertainties of the complex hydraulic fracturing industry and to suggest and even demand that universities invest in research exploring alternative energy technologies.

MULTI-MODALITY AND REPRESENTATION OF TECHNICAL NETWORKS OF ENVIRONMENTAL RISK

In Pennsylvania and Ohio, activists were frustrated that there were no statewide spaces to explore issues of human health effects as a result of the hydraulic fracturing industry. Neither Pennsylvania nor Ohio Departments of Health listed any part of the hydraulic fracturing industry (extraction, storage, or transport) exposure as a concern on their state environmental health data systems. Also, there were no institutionally state-sponsored baseline studies about health and HVHF. However, activists pointed to community groups, like the Center for Coalfield Justice, that linked the risk of known risks (the coal industry) with other extractive practices, like coal mining, which was helpful in networking, particularly along environmental justice arguments in Appalachia in both Pennsylvania and Ohio, for positioning legislation for laws to protect ecosystems and people in them.

While many of the same discourse patterns in Ohio were shared in Pennsylvania, it is important to note when other ideologies challenged various pro-industry frames.

As noted in chapter 2, though not specified on state policy sites, the southeastern area of the state has a different natural storyline related to the Chesapeake Bay that complicates a pro-industry narrative. While the Chesapeake Bay Foundation (CBF) has considerable agency in shaping HVHF policy in the Chesapeake Bay watershed areas in Pennsylvania, other statements made by powerful policy holders, particularly as regards to water in large metro areas, such as Philadelphia, suggest a very different framing of HVHF than pro-industry, as outlined by Finewood and Stroup (2012):

> stakeholders must weigh the potential risks to water against their personal economic welfare, their communities' environmental health, as well as the economic welfare of the nation as a whole. In contrast, opponents of fracking often frame a more complex narrative about water. In this view, not only are local places and associated resources experiencing social, economic, and ecological costs that far outweigh the benefits of natural gas production, stakeholders are (re)framing the protection of water resources in non-economic terms, such as a life-giving resource critical to community values and as a human/non-human right. (e.g., Hope, 2009; Charman, 2010, p. 73)

For example, a page detailing information about HVHF in the Delaware River Basin discusses the Philadelphia Water Department's position concerning HVHF:

> For centuries, the pristine forests of the northern portion of the basin have provided clean water to support Philadelphia and Southeast Pennsylvania's vibrant economy . . . The assurance of a sustainable, clean source of drinking water for our citizens is our pledge for today and for generations to come. ("Marcellus Shale Drilling in the Delaware River Basin")

Here, a new frame, one of sustainability (Dryzek, 2005), uses language that suggests alternatives to simple pro-industry narratives. Phrases like "pristine forests"; "clean water"; "clean source of drinking water" and the inclusive "for our citizens" through an extended time "for today and for generations to come" offers alternatives to the ways in which industry and time were discussed in the previous Ohio example.

Of course, this is only in some parts of the state. Ohio, too, has small communities and public lands that ban HVHF, but not to the extent that larger sections of PA has done so. What is problematic, of course, in both states, are the ways in which already marginalized communities are impacted by HVHF because geographically, other pro-industry frames hold sway.

Ouellette points to the following in terms of social circulation: "the emotional reactions and the circulation that results from those reactions determines, in large part, which amplified messages gain velocity and the kinds of social relations that emerge. Such affective circulation further determines what messages/rhetorics endure" (2017). Similarly, Nixon's scholarship on the ways in which activists might consider "storylines" of how complex, long-term environmental injustices (and intervening justices) might be represented and circulated more widely (2011). In the case of my study, activists routinely cited that social media was often the "entry" into other networked sites and activities that allowed for the formation of "counter" representation of risk with varying agency in each state. More than one activist noted that they had earned a "Masters" or "PhD" in understanding the intricacies of environmental risk. For example, Diane stated that she had spent "hours of (research) . . . I earned a master's degree in fracking." This research was not from simply spending time on social media, but in accessing networks of knowledge that began on environmental Facebook groups or blog posts. Activists noted the extensive time spent understanding the complexity of risk inherent in hydraulic fracturing that was often not represented within institutionalized environmental risk participatory mechanisms by exploring legal documents, mapping (paper and digital), local, state, and federal environmental policy, impacts of chemicals in a variety of contextualized scenarios, air quality, and hazardous waste through all parts of production, including transportation and disposal. Activists kept and shared emerging peer-reviewed studies about HVHF, including databases about research in several scientific disciplines.

New York

New York's effective methods of social circulation involved, before the state ban, establishing "home rule" in many local communities, which gave the local communities the right to regulate industry based on arguments that showcased intersections of HVHF risk. I spoke to New York activist, Sally, who was instrumental in helping to challenge HVHF in the town of Dryden, New York, which was highly covered by the media, including a Bill Moyers and *Mother Jones* profile that was widely shared on social media about the ban, to discover how she framed citizen's rights. It should be noted that Dryden's ban also relied heavily on a complicated zoning law that required two lawyers, who happened to live near the community, who used extensive knowledge of New York law to win the initial and subsequent ban. Their legal arguments have since been referred to within NY legislation and in other states.

Pennsylvania

Additionally, circulation of local representation of risks is important. Tim, who ran the *FracTracker Alliance* site in Pennsylvania discussed the ways in which crowd-sourced pictures of all parts of the industry process that told a tale of the industry that institutional sites did not share, such as

- "air quality concerns,"
- "compressor stations,"
- "disposal sites,"
- "pipelines,"
- "rigs," and
- "water concerns."

The FracTracker site began to organize and categorize risks beyond what institutional sites represented as risks.

Counter-literacy narratives allowed for several multimodal, sophisticated representations of risk shared on community-based risk reporting sites such as the *FracTracker Alliance* site, which re-represents data from state institutional sites, but also uses sites like Google mapping to reveal disclosures of well sites, accidents, spills, and proposed pipelines that are not easily found on easily on state and federal institutional sites. Interfaces on *FracTracker* maps consider feminist geographies[1] to provide risk exploration beyond "permitting" and "regulation" and to more critically interrogate how geographic spatialities of risk are being represented. For example, mapping layers include an "environmental justice" layer to contextualize risks. Some activists found that the crowd-sourced images and video clips of all parts of the industry process shared online tell a tale of risk, again, a narrative, of the industry that institutional sites did not share. According to activists Tim and Sam, the FracTracker Alliance site began to organize and categorize risks beyond what institutional sites represented as risks at all, for example, the inclusion of an "environmental justice" tool as a mapping layer allows users to investigate hydraulic fracking more critically and discusses both institutional and community-based water monitoring efforts. This map includes ways in which institutional sites might define risks across state borders and opens policy deliberations that include ecosystems that do not simply stop at state lines or within state policies: "The dark green outlines are in PA only and contain oil and gas summaries of wells and violations. The light green outlines show agency-based monitoring activity and are not restricted to PA boundaries. The reason for the two layers is that states classify oil and gas wells differently and so cannot be combined easily."

Finally, multi-modality allows for the representation of what material feminist and ecofeminist scholars recognize as the relationship of the flux between the human body and material surroundings. Alaimo (2007) refers to this notion as "trans-corporeal feminism" and suggests such understandings of materials and bodies contribute significantly to understandings of culture by pointing to the complicated ways in which bodies in space become marginalized through toxins created from socio-cultural constructions. "As a particularly vivid example of trans-corporeal space, toxic bodies insist that environmentalism, human health and social justice cannot be severed. They encourage us to imagine ourselves in constant interchange with the 'environment'" (p. 262). Alaimo discusses a complex web of intersectional chemical contamination that "poisons the workers who produce it, the neighborhood in which it is produced, and the plants and animals who end up consuming it" and points to varied but connected inquiries into this contamination: "the traffic in toxins reveals interconnections between various movements, such as those of environmental health, occupational health, labor movements, environmental justice, environmentalism, ecological medicine, disability rights, green living, anti-globalization, consumer rights, and child welfare" (2007, p. 260).

Material feminist theory underscores how, in my study, activists found ways to represent complex intersectional fracking industry results on and within organisms: land, and human bodies and the human social systems that promote such industrial activities. Often, these photos and videos of material risks were shared between activists in cyberspace, but through images, powerful material risk circulated. The results of earthquakes on properties (cracked foundations) were shared among activists long before the Department of Natural Resources in Ohio formally made a formal and official link between injection wells (that store hydraulic fracturing waste) and earthquakes. Maps of trains carrying hazardous materials through densely populated neighborhoods and schools shifted conversations about what officials claimed was the "safe" transport and disposal of HVHF waste. Images of children with nosebleeds by those living near hydraulic fracturing compressor stations in

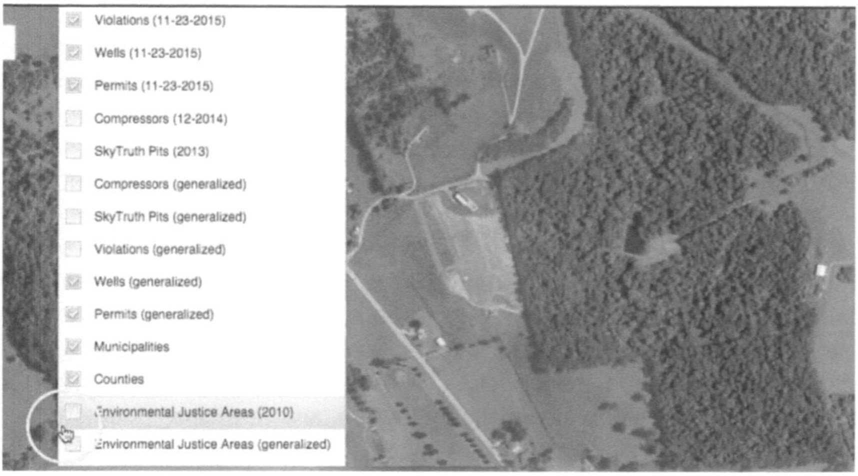

Figure 3.1 Environmental Justice Mapping Layer. *Source*: Screenshot by author.

several states were widely shared to advance networks of inquiry into possible connections between public health and hydraulic fracturing. Several of the activists I interviewed had been arrested at some point (often, fines to pay for arrests were crowd-sourced through online community groups), so they were familiar with ways that their material bodies became sites of protest and deliberation, however unsanctioned at the time.

Again, as suggested earlier in this chapter, where state institutions fail, activist groups like the FracTracker Alliance combine information from Pennsylvania institutional sites and publicly available tools like Google Maps to provide visuals that show intersectional concerns, such as seen in figure 3.1 from Shelly's TAP, where Environmental Justice areas and HVHF are visually layered, offering an "Environmental Justice" mapping layer on mapping tools from Google Maps and PA institutional sites:

Shelly explained that the figure 3.1 is also connected to Google Earth mapping, which displays mapping with contextual features, so activists can see varied map images, a simple tool linked to free and open source data.

> If you click on it . . . Fractracker does explains exactly what this is . . . so click on it, and then, the base map . . . . it links to Google earth images too, so I can just do that [clicks] . . . this is the feature I love the most. You just type your address in and it takes you right there. So now I can see my house. If I want to know about this gas well I can just literally click on it and read what it is.

As this example displays, the accessibility of varied mapping layer tools that show the HVHF industry is important in risk representation.

Additionally, because of the environmental justice concerns that arose from decades of coal industry, activist groups like the Center for Coalfield Justice were able to publish and make available to public stakeholders a baseline report entitled "Community Indicators of Environmental Justice" that provided a systematic look at a variety of intersectional concerns. Titled "Community Indicators," this report on Greene and Washington counties in southeastern Pennsylvania juxtaposed coal mining, shale drilling, population growth, birth rate, mortality, natural increase, dependent population (under 18 over 65), land areas and population density, race, cases of abuse per 1000 children, crime rates, housing values, homeownership, vacancies, public school dropout rate, federal expenditures, household income, income source, unemployment, employment sectors, poverty rate, public school revenue, cash and medical public assistance, highways, and farmland—among other indicators, to provide a wider discussion of the impacts of industry in these areas. Though not official state policy (HVHF is widely practiced in the area), this work is a testament to the ways in which communities collect information that may increase agency as HVHF is more widely studied . . . and as its risks are more clearly understood. This proactive approach suggests "Ecological Democracy" language frames that many suggest should be more widely considered, particularly in already marginalized spaces (Dryzek, 2005). However, such distinctions are not a part of Pennsylvania's institutionalized HVHF public deliberation process. Perhaps what is most noteworthy about the ideologies embedded in these texts is the focus on "industry" and the pattern of permitting for industry.

It should be noted that such an environmental justice approach, though compelling, often not successful as laws regulating hydraulic fracturing simply have yet to be written, and further studies about the various impacts of hydraulic fracturing have yet to be funded and carried out.

However, in each state, experts/activists in the medical field worked to provide such information to the public, and these works were widely shared among activists. For example, in Pennsylvania, the Southwest Pennsylvania Environmental Health Project provides online resources and health services and monitoring of human bodies and equipment to monitor air quality to those living near HVHF gas wells. In Ohio, the Center for Health, Environment and Justice, again, not affiliated with a state agency, provides a "Prevent Fracking Harms" page with links to resources about health effects, including a database about emerging health studies, grounded in a recognition of possible embodied risks of this industry, and contextualizing risk in local environments and in local bodies.

By comparison, the Southwest Pennsylvania Environmental Health Project positions itself very differently from institutional resources explored above in that it more closely aligns itself with intersectional environmental justice approaches. These patterns offer a possibility for depicting risk through technical communication poised for environmental action. As noted earlier in this chapter, the mission is stated as follows: "The Environmental Health Project (EHP) is a nonprofit public health organization that assists and supports residents of Southwest Pennsylvania and beyond who believe their health has been, or could be, impacted by unconventional oil and gas development (UOGD, or fracking)." (Southwest Pennsylvania Environmental Health Project, 2021, About). More so than any of the previous sites, this group offers an unequivocal description of health risk related to HVHF.

The question at the bottom of stasis, *Are there health risks related to HVHF?* Is answered with a firm yes. Not only does the Southwest Pennsylvania Environmental Health Project assert that there are health risks they note that the risks are "substantial."

Unlike the other sites which limited discussion of health issues related to HVHF, links to intersecting types of health risks in detailing specific types of health concerns from different parts of HVHF industry are linked to emerging research, answering the definitional level of stasis: *What are the health risks?* There are embedded and separate resource links to academic, community, and nonprofit studies about HVHF environmental health risks that enable a scholarly discussion in response to this question, which is part of the *is* level of stasis.

Definitions of risk are much more clear and specific than in the previous regulatory and advisory institutional websites, where risks were framed as "uncertain" and "monitored" by institutional experts. Instead, the Southwest PA Environmental Health Project includes researched details of how air quality, water quality, noise and light, stress, and soil as impacted by HVHF also impact human bodies.

Also, there is a temporal element, as health risks are delineated as short-term and long-term effects that are a result of the contextualized HVHF industry. For example, in the "air quality" section, there are details about how the different parts of HVHF contribute to issues of human health. The accompanying research, found throughout the page, backs the assertions for each area of concern and research projects through various institutions with whom EHP collaborated.

There are several jurisdiction suggestions based on the lower *stasis (Should there be action based on health risks? What is the action suggested based on what authority?).* The Southwest PA Environmental Health projects make many suggestions based on values of environmental justice and "green politics." For example, for each area of environmental concern, there are short-term and long-term suggestions so citizens can self-monitor for the area of concern, creating a nuanced and "layered" understanding of risk and promoting agency for public participants in contributing to risk reporting about:

- Air Quality
- Water Quality
- Noise and Light
- Stress
- Soil
- Emergency Preparedness

NARRATIVE REPRESENTATIONS OF ENVIRONMENTAL RISK

In addition to social circulation, activist interviews revealed patterns of narrative within their inquiry. Narratives offer important spaces for environmental risk deliberation scholarship, and composition studies are helpful to understand both the limitations and agency narratives might provide. As writing studies scholar Debra Journet notes, "narratives are still being written against the grain of academic discourse." Journet asks us to consider personal narrative, but to also consider, more clearly, "genred narratives" and how historically, the validity of narratives that "correspond to the reality of the phenomena under discussion" (2012, p. 19). At issue with hydraulic fracturing are the competing narratives of risk, and how agency is given to particular narratives. While public comment (if offered) might allow activists to discuss personal, anecdotal experiences in a public setting, scholarship suggests these narratives, even if revealing localized phenomena of risk, often do not have much agency in the traditional top-down approach to environmental risk decision-making; thus, sharing a personal narrative is often not part of true environmental "deliberation." However, among activists, narratives propel new ways of considering environmental risk, challenging the positioning of "regulation" of an industry by experts backing industrial science without widespread scientific precautionary studies. Journet challenges writing studies scholars to think more critically about *how* personal narratives might or might not be privileged in a particular situation. In my study, narratives allowed activists to share personal experiences among themselves that were not being represented by regulatory institutions—and allowed for participants to more fully adopt a sense of identity in terms of "sharing a place at the table." Shared narratives such as those in *Shalefield Stories: A Project of Friends of the Harmed* allowed activists to respond with support, in immediate ways, to those who could not afford, in terms of money and time, for the institutional regulatory to make reparations about possible material environmental damage—to the living organisms (including people) within ecological systems which activists contend were affected by hydraulic fracturing. Narratives allowed activists to contextualize highly technical risk information, such as the information represented on the *FracTracker Alliance* site, which combines technical data from institutional sites with narrative within multimodal digital storytelling formats.

At times, a narrative might be effective in that it offers a different technical frame from what an institutional site might offer. For example, the details of risks of an ethane cracker plant[2] in Western PA became more widely known by framing risks beyond the Pennsylvania Department of Environmental Protection sites offered. Information about risks on FracTracker comes from state regulatory sites but is formatted in understandable language and also includes counter narratives that state regulations tend to leave out. For example, FracTracker Alliance lists limitations of current evacuation plans and disclosures of the distances between the cracker plant and hospitals, schools, and population size, bringing to light who might be impacted by the cracker plant.

Similarly, FracTracker Alliance shares, along with the narrative of the risks of the cracker plant, an alternative to the industry narrative often heard in public meetings (and largely difficult to navigate to or absent on institutional sites) by introducing environmental right-to-know and environmental justice rights, as well as attendant mapping of Environmental Justice communities (EJ) near the cracker plant. This awareness of possible personal agency links to my previous statements about the ways in which activists in localities such as Dryden or Ohio might become key players in making decisions about environmental risk.

Additionally, the marginalization of Pennsylvania's landscape have given rise to some local advocacy groups like the Southwest Pennsylvania Environmental Health Project, which tells a different narrative about environmental risk. The EHP defines itself as follows: "The Environmental Health Project (EHP) is a nonprofit public health organization that assists and supports residents of Southwestern Pennsylvania and beyond who believe their health has been, or could be, impacted by unconventional oil and gas development (UOGD, or fracking)" (Southwest Environmental Health Project, 2021, About EHP) who seek a concerted public health response in spite of "the lack of objective, reliable data on the health effects of UOGD activities raises many questions about the origins of residents' health problems and the scope of public health risks in communities" (Southwest Environmental Health Project, 2021, About EHP). Another important note is that due to the Halliburton Loophole in the Energy Act of 2005, mentioned previously in this chapter, these SMCRA regulations do not apply to HVHF drilling or storage operations, sparking a concern by many stakeholders about intersectional or layered risks of multiple industries through space and time. In an ironic twist, there are many places in Pennsylvania where HVHF operations exist beside or within acid mine drainage restoration sites. The lack of "precautionary" language within deliberations for supposedly "clean" innovations like HVHF means toxic, carbon-based industries will continue. Pennsylvania's environmental identity is deeply entwined with its history of energy extraction, but the geographic distribution of risk is clustered in the northeastern through the southwestern parts of the state, partly dictated by the way in which the possible recoverable shale gas is in the southwestern and northeastern parts of the state.

Here, I argue that it is in analyzing ways in which the *is* is defined by various actors in HVHF risk that leads to understanding the ways socially situated assumptions of values often appear in discussions of risk, and, by extension, the *ought*, of the HVHF policies and practices informed by these definitions (Schiappa, 1998), particularly in locales like Southwestern PA with a deep extractive history. It is the discrepancy between the "is" and the "ought" that leads to different definitions of risks, and different policies and practices that can be applied across language used by various stakeholders, making narratives about the right to health difficult.

The Southwest Pennsylvania Environmental Health Project positions itself very differently from institutional resources like the Pennsylvania Health Department, which does not account for HVHF is a variable for risks to human health. The Southwest Pennsylvania Environmental Health Project more closely aligns itself with narratives of intersectional environmental justice approaches. These patterns offer a possibility for depicting risk through technical communication poised for environmental action. As noted earlier in this chapter, the mission is stated as follows: "The Environmental Health Project (EHP) is a nonprofit public health organization that assists and supports residents of Southwest Pennsylvania and beyond who believe their health has been, or could be, impacted by unconventional oil and gas development (UOGD, or fracking)." (Southwest Pennsylvania Environmental Health Project, 2021, About). More so than any of the previous sites, this group offers an unequivocal description of health risk related to HVHF.

The question at the bottom of stasis, *Are there health risks related to HVHF?* Is answered with a firm yes. Not only does the Southwest Pennsylvania Environmental Health Project assert that there are health risks; they note that the risks are "substantial" as noted from lines from their site: "Data suggests that unconventional oil and gas development (UOGD or 'fracking') poses substantial risk to public health from the toxic chemicals used during the industrial process, as well as from other associated problems" (Southwest PA Environmental Health Project, 2021).

Unlike the other institutional sites which limited discussion of health issues related to HVHF, links to intersecting types of health risks, detailing specific types of health concerns from different parts of the HVHF industry are linked to emerging research, answering the definitional level of stasis: *What are the health risks?* There are embedded and separate resource links to academic, community, and nonprofit studies about HVHF environmental health risks that enable a scholarly discussion in response to this question, which is part of the *is* level of stasis. An excerpt from the site highlights several intersecting risks:

> Research is mounting on the emissions from UOGD at all stages and on health effects experienced by nearby residents. Many of the toxic chemicals that have been found in air and water samples around UOGD operations have well known adverse health effects. For example, benzene is a known carcinogen (cancer-causing), toluene is a neurotoxin, and hydrogen sulfide irritates the lungs and can cause asthma. Noise and light pollution is associated with hearing loss, sleeplessness, and other health issues. (Southwest PA Environmental Health Project, 2021, Health Issues)

Definitions of risk are much more clear and specific than in the previous regulatory and advisory institutional websites, where risks were framed as "uncertain" and "monitored" by institutional experts. Instead, the Southwest PA Environmental Health Project includes researched details of how air quality, water quality, noise and light, stress, and soil as impacted by HVHF also impact human bodies.

Also, there is a temporal element, as health risks are delineated as short-term and long-term effects that are a result of the contextualized HVHF industry. For example, in the "air quality" section, there are details about how research has found that different parts of HVHF contribute to issues of human health such as short-term effects: "burning eyes, sore throat, stomach pain and nausea, headaches, and tingling/numbness in the extremities" in addition to long-term effects "from pollution such as cancer, cardiovascular disease, and poor birth outcomes" (Southwest PA Environmental Health Project, 2021, Health Issues).

The accompanying research, found throughout the page, backs the assertions for each area of concern and research projects through various institutions with whom EHP collaborated.

There are several jurisdiction suggestions based on the lower stasis *(Should there be action based on health risks? What is the action suggested based on what authority?).* The Southwest PA Environmental Health projects make many suggestions based on values of environmental justice and "green politics." For example, for each area of environmental concern, there are short-term and long-term suggestions so citizens can self-monitor for the area of concern, creating a nuanced and "layered" understanding of risk and promoting agency for public participants in contributing to risk reporting—these include "air and water quality, noise and light, soil, and emergency preparedness." Also, participants are actively asked to report risks, inviting stakeholder knowledge into the risk-making process.

Within the links, such as the "Air Quality" link, there are instructions about the use of simple tools such as Purple Air monitors that link to a larger community-based Community Science Project to monitor air quality rather than waiting for an expert to monitor it for them. There are also tips for practical steps stakeholders can take at home to reduce air quality concerns, as well as links to resources so concerned stakeholders can understand the cause and effect of HVHF and the specific health concern or even to stakeholders' identities: parents, HVHF employees, medical professionals, etc. Finally, stakeholders can link to legal advice, other nonprofit community groups researching environmental health risk as related to HVHF, environmental reporting links for potential hazards such as spills or other violations, emergency planning tips, including directions for filing a right-to-know request and instructions about attending Local Emergency Planning Committees and asking questions about chemicals.

There is also a section for health care providers, including continuing education for those working in HVHF industries and links to professional groups that routinely investigate the link between HVHF and public health concerns.

Throughout the site, it is clear that a green politics ideology is the main narrative, which values intersectional environmental justice principles, offers direction for agency for individual stakeholders living near HVHF activity, often linking various activist groups. Nature is seen as a complex ecosystem, and complex interactions between humans and the natural world, especially as related to HVHF, are acknowledged.

However, what is surprising on this site is the lack of discussion to halt HVHF and precautionary language that limits HVHF. One of the action items highlighted at the level of jurisdiction (ought) is that of "set back distances," which recommend HVHF activity exist further away from humans.

In a sense, this is a reactionary approach (the HVHF activity will continue, but the suggestion is that it does so further away from human residences). However, despite calls for links between health risks and HVHF, there is little information about banning HVHF on the premise that there are likely many unknown health risks. This could be because the Southwest PA Environmental Health Project exists in an area that has a long history of extractive resources that are part of the geographical "identity," which helps to maintain HVHF as a status quo activity in the area. As noted earlier in this chapter, New York health officials continue to take a much stronger stance in their approach to HVHF activity, repeatedly reiterating that the entire industry is fraught with human health risks.

NOTES

1. Feminist geography, according to Moss and Falconer Al-Hindi (2000), attends to issues of authority (both claiming and contesting authority) and power in terms of representing spatial phenomena. In my study, feminist geography's attention to spatial representation, particularly representing those that have been marginalized, is crucial as feminist geographers grapple with critical issues of representing spatial social inequality.

2. Cracker plants convert Natural Gas Liquids (NGLs), which are products of the HVHF, to energy ("What is a Cracker," 2017).

Chapter 4

Linguistic Frames

Stories of Environmental Activism, New York, Changing Policy, and Practice

One of the most compelling examples of different types of social constructs of risk is the case study of New York. As noted earlier, activists were successful in implementing an HVHF drilling ban by linking discussions to green discourse and storylines that include environmental justice and intersectional and precautionary discourses.

Social media allowed activists to learn about and participate in activist events, including coordinating public comment sponsored by local, state, and federal institutions, and events opposing the limitations of such institutions. For example, participants from the "We Are Seneca Lake" activist group, who opposed natural gas storage under Seneca Lake in existing salt caverns from past industry, offered a variety of ways to encourage dialogue about possible risks by organizing their website along the lines of providing informational (access to press releases, media, video, brochures, and newsletters), access to community (by becoming a Seneca Lake Defender), and action (by engaging in petitions and letters to elected officials) (Lovejoy and Saxton, 2012). Samuel discussed how the website provides access to letter writing campaigns to elected officials and access to scientific studies, particularly those completed by non-industry scientists. Additionally, Participant 4 detailed the usability of the site for organizing and documenting complex deliberations about risk:

> It's got an emphasis on public outreach, ease of access, a lot of pictures . . . press releases . . . everything this group does gets videotaped . . . we have a videographer who comes to almost every protest, every court hearing.

Samuel also detailed an arrest campaign, noting a tab that, when selected, showed resources that invited users to explore what it meant to go to jail, the procedures for nonviolent arrest, funding contributions for a defense fund for those arrested, and a good deal of thought given to planned groups for strategic arrest: elaborating that "teachers" and "people of faith" each had specialized "arrest" weeks (among others) to highlight the notion of participants as community members versus members simply presenting themselves as "radical activists." Samuel outlined an increase in arrests that occurred after the positioning of the NY activists toward arrest as civil disobedience after FERC (Federal Energy Regulatory Commission) approved more methane gas storage under Seneca Lake without meaningful public comment consideration about potential risks: "We have no other recourse . . . that's when these folks decided to get arrested . . . People are willing to say, 'I am going to be arrested'—I had never been arrested before." Activists found that civil disobedience, including arrests, was an integral part of risk communication within environmental injustices. Communicating environmental messages, including linking environmental activism to "civil disobedience," was crucial for activist groups.

An important theme that many activists shared was their legality in terms of their right to access risk information and the way in which resisting risk was often criminalized—and how resisting this criminalization became an important narrative. Most of the activists I spoke to had been arrested at one point, and telling their narratives of arrest in terms of "civil disobedience" of what they felt to be an unjust energy regime was an important part of their emerging identity as an activist. Several of my participants were part of the "Seneca Lake Defenders" group, who identified as "defending" human and ecological rights. They took turns, over a series of years, blockading an industrial access site for gas storage under Seneca Lake and were often arrested for this action. The defenders took pains to identify as environmental heroes (thus, the term "defenders" versus criminals). The arrests were well-organized, including planning who might be arrested at a given time, press releases surrounding arrests, and extensive legal and financial assistance to those who were arrested. Accompanying many of the arrests are narratives that critique the lack of precaution for the gas storage plan, concern about climate change, lack of industry oversight, and encouragement of renewable energy. Activists clearly felt a sense of "community" and, perhaps, "heroism" in nonviolent civil disobedience among these actions, which can be seen in the introduction to the arrests page:

> There are hundreds of Seneca Lake Defenders. These are the faces of people who have been arrested after using nonviolent civil disobedience to stand up against Crestwood. Here's what they have to say about why they are willing to risk arrest:

> 657 arrests have been made at the gates of Crestwood since the We Are Seneca Lake campaign began. 404 different Seneca Lake Defenders have been arrested. In addition, at least 144 Seneca Lake Defenders have successfully blockaded for an entire day without being arrested. ("The Seneca Lake Defenders")

June, an active participant from New York, wrote and published a narrative of her arrest in a local literary magazine that detailed the tensions of being a mother and her arrest, discussing her value system in which she felt the need to protect her child's future outweighed the social stigma of an arrest.[1]

POST-POSITIVIST NOTIONS OF SCIENCE: JUSTICE AND PRECAUTION—CONSIDERING PUBLIC HEALTH

Several of the activists I have met in my study are involved in persuasive performances in highly technical and complex rhetorical spaces. For example, some shared highly technical information about solar or wind technologies that might act as alternative infrastructures for communities. Other stakeholders involved in "citizen science" initiatives are taking active roles in complex, technical, but often localized, scientific studies (Jasanoff, 2003; Conrad and Hilchey, 2011) to study air or water. But what was noteworthy was the way in which networks of agency invoked when activists investigated issues of public health. These notions of localized sciences within shared networks created knowledge in proactive ways. It is important here to discuss theoretical frameworks about this kind of contextualized science information. Functowicz and Ravetz (1993) consider the way in which socially constructed notions of uncertainty complicates past "normal" positivist science philosophies. Within these systems, powerful new ideologies can be brought to light, with which activists engaged: in this case, environmental justice and decisions based on the precautionary principle are feminist in terms of a call for ecological democracy, situated in a critique of cultural constructs that lead to the marginalization of ecologies and organisms, including people, in them (Dryzek, 2005). Frameworks of environmental justice that explore discursive possibilities attending to expanded notions of citizen risk reporting in space and time (Holifield, Porter, and Walker, 2010). Environmental justice attends to resituating discourse about environmental risks due to "the legacy of a disproportionate burden imposed on poor and minority communities by environmental harmful conditions, [and calls for] more inclusive opportunities for those who are most affected to be heard in the decisions made by public agencies" (Cox, 2006, p. 290). Environmental justice frameworks seek more complex ideas about how places are labeled for industrial practices and how those living in geographically stigmatized spaces, as defined by dominant discourses, might find agency in redefining place, and, by extension, personal identity. Here, Jacqueline Schiappa's articulation of "intersectionality" provides a more complex representation of oppressions: "the fact that many social groups experience oppression along *multiple* planes, and second, that those planes are conceptually and materially *inseparable*" (2017, in press). This acknowledgment of layers of oppression through time and space is crucial to understand in terms of the silencing of activists through largely ineffective institutional public comment that does not consider the complex marginalizations activists feel: there are cumulative issues of air quality, water quality, soil quality, seismic issues, and long-term economic quality that are not often included in deliberations. Added to this, these fracking activities often occur near locations of economic poverty that do not have resources to represent these varied risks.

Similarly, ideologies of precautionary politics suggest that in complex and uncertain environmental issues, where scientific consensus cannot or has not been reached, the public should not bear the burden of "proving" risks as is currently the case; publics, instead, should be protected if a reasonable risk has been found (Whiteside, 2006). By adopting environmental justice and precautionary ideologies, both feminist in nature, activists were able to challenge normate views of the environment as a "resource" that fulfills a dominant economic narrative, and to call for more rigorous and expanded scientific studies.

Environmental justice, intersectionality, and precautionary frames are useful for spurring new knowledge making, which was widely represented and shared in the technical reading and writing practices of activists. Activists networked outside of localities to represent risks not sanctioned by institutional environments in their own states.

INTERVENTIONS: COUNTER-LITERACIES LEADING TO A NEW YORK BAN ON HVHF

Simmons and Grabill's (2007) research on communities accessing technology to "invent" and "perform persuasively" valued knowledge given a complex rhetorical situation related to environmental deliberation dovetails nicely with the New York activists I encountered in my study (2007, p. 422). Interestingly, one resource included on the Ohio site Center for Health, Environment and Justice page links to several of New York's deliberations about the decisions to ban fracking in New York State, highlighting the networking that occurs among activists that I observed during my interviews and think-aloud protocols. The New York State ban on high-volume hydraulic fracturing acts as a literate artifact, of sorts; in many ways, it is the end result of interactions between grassroots activists and experts in many states sharing and compiling information challenging an industrial "norm" of hydraulic fracturing. Many activists in my study contributed to knowledge building that resulted in a state-wide ban: sharing studies about emerging health issues in places like Pennsylvania and Ohio, such as the online narratives collected on the *List of the Harmed* site, which collects narratives of medical harms to ecosystems, humans, and animals caused by HVHF chemicals.

New York activists collected this knowledge, building political and legal cases for bans in various communities, then networking successes to state-wide discussions of the practice. It is important to note that prior to the ban, activists were assured by officials from the New York Department of Conservation that the HVHF industry could be regulated and that spills and accidents were extremely rare. However, activists in New York traveled to neighboring states of Ohio and Pennsylvania and witnessed the results of explosions, water contamination, and methane leaks. Their "felt" sense of risk, and conversations with their neighbors' perceptions of risk did not match up to the "institutionalized" representations of risk. The Dimock, PA water case (easily accessible to New York), in which the industry denied that HVHF caused widespread water contamination to private property in the Dimock area, generated investigations by activists into both "knowledge making" about risk in Pennsylvania, but also about how risks might be averted in New York through fracking bans. Across the state of New York, anti-fracking activists attended public meetings and flooded local and state public comment. The New York activists I spoke to discussed networks of knowledge that supported this grassroots movement: how to write letters to local, state, and federal representatives, how to navigate legal issues to impose industry bans in local areas (culminating in a "home-rule" orientation which allowed local governments, not the state, to control how drilling might occur, if it occurred at all), and how to read and represent highly technical information from emerging scholarly studies about environmental and public health risks. In response to the perceived lack of true deliberation about potential risks, many New York activists turned to the "body" as a form of speech. Their "bodies" spoke through marches, blockades, and arrests, and these experiences and rationales for them were widely shared online. Several activists I interviewed shared information on how to commit acts of civil disobedience, using literate networks to plan who and how to be arrested; groups also coordinated fundraising to pay fines and legal representation for arrested activists. While activists in Ohio and Pennsylvania employed similar tactics, it was the reaction in New York to what had happened in the nearby states that created a large community-based outcry against what activists felt were very real risks in the HVHF industry. The ban on the extractive practice of hydraulic fracking occurred in December of 2014. In June of 2015, the New

York Department of Environmental Conservation (DEC) announced the following: "The SEQR Findings Statement for high-volume hydraulic fracturing (HVHF) was issued on June 29, 2015. This concluded DEC's comprehensive, seven-year review and officially prohibits HVHF in New York." This page, as earlier noted, is situated within the DEC site and takes some navigating to find, but does offer acknowledgment of the public comments that helped to shape the way risks were investigated, including a prioritization of public health not represented in the Ohio or Pennsylvania institutional sites, where HVHF drilling is still legal. This page, as earlier noted, is situated within the site and takes some navigating to find, but does offer acknowledgment of the public review and public comments that helped to shape the way risks were investigated, including a prioritization on both public comment and public health not represented in the Ohio or Pennsylvania institutional sites.

While the New York Department of Environmental Conservation puts some authority for this decision in the hands of the New York State Department of Health, a longer statement refers to a rare, meaningful interaction between the public and a state agency to create knowledge about risk. It is clear here that questions of "value" have been represented, at the insistence of citizens, beyond the expertise of regulation of an industry. Expertise in public health is represented in this decision. While activists in New York were pleased with these successes, they noted the opposition they faced in attempting to articulate this aspect of risk. The entire deliberation centered on citizens and experts proving that there was enough risk to warrant the statewide ban. The activists still currently face deliberations about the transport and storage of gas, which are still hotly contested throughout the state as transportation infrastructure for HVHF continues in light of gas exports.

As discussed earlier in this book, participants in all locations felt the frustration of having to "prove" HVHF risks over time against the positioning of industry not responsible for a longer time period than industry extraction. They were frustrated by the way in which the pro-industry position is simply exempt from recognizing complex risk in terms of precaution in terms of HVHF: "The precautionary principle applies especially in situations of environmental risk where by the time unambiguous scientific evidence of a serious problem becomes available, the danger may have already have materialized and perhaps become irreversible" (viii, Whiteside, 2006, p. viii). Many participants vocalized a particular concern when noting intersectional risks that might be compounded by time which are often not represented on most institutional regulatory sites. For example, participants in Ohio were particularly concerned about the intersections of seismic activity, water, radioactivity, soil contamination, and property values over time. These possible compounded risks simply don't have "definitional" purchase for possible policy and action. This becomes even more of a concern as much of

HVHF activity occurs in spaces that have suffered a "slow violence" from past industrial cycles (Nixon, 2011).

Because all participants voiced frustration over the lack of precautionary language in institutional risk participatory mechanisms, it is illuminating to compare the notion of "precaution" between states that have banned HVHF drilling and those who have not. New York, for example, does not ban all industrial portions of HVHF activity, but does ban the practice of HVHF drilling, partly by discussing possible negative health effects from unknown risks by shifting agency. All participants from all states were aware of the New York ban based on a public health argument, so it is helpful to explore that move.

During Samuel's TAP, he discussed a Supplemental Generic *Environmental Impact* Statement (SGEIS) on a New York Department of Environmental Conservation site that he had been following online.[2] New York was the only state that offered an Environmental Impact Report. As noted earlier in this chapter and in chapter 3, Samuel discussed the difficulties most public participants would have in accessing the environmental impact report (which was, according to Samuel, positioned to explore and to promote HVHF activity in the state) but suggested that many did so, resulting in an unprecedented number of public comments.

Within this SGEIS, which in itself was positioned *for* HVHF activity by framing HVHF in line with past, more benign drilling activities, Samuel navigated to a Department of Health statement that largely provided the rationale for the HVHF drilling ban in the state of New York. Samuel discussed the deliberation process, including unprecedented public comment mentioned in a link from the SGEIS. Public comment prompted more public hearings and more comments, including comments on proposed additions to HVHF regulations. The discussion of public participation in regards to HVHF is rare on an institutional site, but, as Samuel pointed out, there is reference to the complexity of the knowledge in regards to varied expert claims: "[as] the volume of new information on HVHF grew, the scope of the review expanded to broadly consider the health impacts of HVHF." In my research, this is one of the few acknowledgments of HVHF as complex and intersecting risks on any state site (and was not readily apparent on the New York Department of Environmental Conservation site).

While Samuel discussed the impact of a report, written by several public health experts and released by a public health expert, Dr. Zucker, he did not navigate to it himself during his TAP; I did so later. Samuel, however, was very clear in terms of highlighting the impact of the report (which was written as a result of increasing public concern, inquiry, and commentary) which effectively pushed for a final SGEIS as released through the NY DEC and ultimately halted HVHF drilling activity in the state of New York. Again, as all participants were aware of the New York HVHF ban based on a public health argument, I felt that the letter is important to review in my research.

My own navigation found that The New York Department of Conservation refers to the report, written by health experts and introduced by NY State Acting Commissioner of Health, Howard Zucker, which was positioned to provide a review of possible human health risks associated with HFHV activity (see table 4.1). It is in this introductory letter that I focus on ideologies within language not often seen on institutional sites: Dryzek terms this ideology "green politics" (2005, p. 218). This discourse includes precautionary, environmental justice, and intersectional approaches.

In assessing Dr. Zucker's introductory letter in terms of green politics discourse, it is clear that the introductory letter positions future HVHF in regards to "unknowns" as a possible risk. As such, this document is listed on the NYDEC page as one of the pieces of evidence to account for the ban of HVHF in New York. Within this letter, the language reveals an ideology very different from administrative and economic rationalization in that it frames public health as criteria for a standard of judgment for HVHF risk. The acknowledgment of a health study itself is an environmental justice concern, showing the study of health as part of the complicated nature of social, economic, and political structures.

Here, Zucker includes suggestions of cumulative effects of industry over time as an important part of establishing criteria. As such, precautionary language (Dryzek, 2005) is seen throughout the letter (see table 4.2). In the following underlined portions of the text, it is clear that a rationale for deciding whether to allow HVHF drilling cannot be completed until time was provided for academic study because of an acknowledgment of complex ecological systems: "This required an evaluation of the emerging scientific information on environmental public health and community health effects." Similarly,

Table 4.1 Green Politics Discourse

Green Politics Story Line *(Dryzek, 2005, p. 218)*
I. Basic entities recognized or constructed (informing ideology)
Global limits
Nature as complex ecosystems
Humans with broad capacities
Social, economic, and political structures
II. Assumptions about natural relationships
Equality among people
Complex interconnections between humans and nature
Subordination of nature
/II. Agents and their motives
Many individual and collective actors, multidimensional motivation
Agency in nature downplayed though not necessarily denied.

complex relationships between humans and nature and the acknowledgment of social, economic, and political structures are invoked in a call for time needed for an analysis of emerging information and existing risk mitigation procedures:

> *This also required an analysis of whether such information was sufficient to determine the extent of potential public health impacts of HVHF activities in New York State (NYS) and whether existing mitigation measures implemented in other states are effectively reducing the risk for adverse public health impacts.*

Similarly, while the complexity of the rhetorical task is noted, the phrases underlined in the excerpt below highlight the linguistic patterns that show uncertainty and the positioning of authority of health risk within scientific studies in accord with existing mitigation possibilities, which legitimizes a precautionary approach to complex and intersecting uncertainties and leads to an HVHF ban. This ban is noteworthy in that unlike all other representations

Table 4.2 Green Politics Discourse, NY Department of Public Health Letter

Dear Commissioner Martens:

It became clear during this assessment that DOH's Public Health Review needed to extend beyond the scope of the initial request to consider, more broadly, the current state of science regarding HVHF and public health risks. This required an evaluation of the emerging scientific information on environmental public health and community health effects. This also required an analysis of whether such information was sufficient to determine the extent of potential public health impacts of HVHF activities in New York State (NYS) and whether existing mitigation measures implemented in other states are effectively reducing the risk for adverse public health impacts.

As with most complex human activities in modern societies, absolute scientific certainty regarding the relative contributions of positive and negative impacts of HVHF on public health is unlikely to ever be attained. In this instance, however, the overall weight of the evidence from the cumulative body of information contained in this Public Health Review demonstrates that there are significant uncertainties about the kinds of adverse health outcomes that may be associated with HVHF, the likelihood of the occurrence of adverse health outcomes, and the effectiveness of some of the mitigation measures in reducing or preventing environmental impacts which could adversely affect public health. Until the science provides sufficient information to determine the level of risk to public health from HVHF to all New Yorkers and whether the risks can be adequately managed, DOH recommends that HVHF should not proceed in NYS.

I appreciate the opportunity to conduct this Public Health Review. It furthers the long history of close collaboration between the two Departments carrying out our shared responsibility to protect human health and the environment.

in this study, the burden of proof lies within proving HVHF mitigation measures are not harmful to public participants vs. public participants[3] proving environmental risk, as can be seen in the following lines:

> *There are significant uncertainties about the kinds of adverse health outcomes* that may be associated with HVHF, *the likelihood of the occurrence of adverse health outcomes, and the effectiveness of some of the mitigation measures in reducing or preventing environmental impacts which could adversely affect public health.* Until the *science provides sufficient information to determine the level of risk to public health* from HVHF to all New Yorkers and whether the risks can be adequately managed, *DOH recommends that HVHF should not proceed in NYS.*

Similarly, the letter ends with a nod to the acknowledgment of complex relationships between humans and nature that might be deliberated through collective actors: "*It furthers the long history of close collaboration between the two Departments carrying out our shared responsibility to protect human health and the environment.*"

While New York participants were pleased with the move to ban HVHF drilling, they all identified that this only banned one aspect of HVHF activity, and all were involved in activist activities that involved transportation and storage issues in New York State. Also, New York participants found that precautionary language was still very rare on the New York DEC pages.

This letter, compared to other representative samples, reveals social constructs (and ideologies that inform social constructs) of possible risks that are unevenly applied across the three states and are revealed in environmental risk participatory mechanisms. This unevenness was keenly felt by participants across states, leading participants to seek alternatives to risk participation in an effort to illuminate risks within the HVHF industry.

This research reveals socially situated constraints and affordances surrounding risk mechanisms that activist participants navigate in an effort to represent environmental risk as related to the HVHF industry. When activists were stymied in deliberation while using institutional environmental risk participatory mechanisms, they turned to various counter-literacies to represent HVHF environmental risk; in the case of New York, these counter-literacies expanded notions of HVHF risk and impacted New York environmental policy in terms of the HVHF drilling ban. I make two arguments based on my data. One is that public access to meaningful deliberation about HVHF environmental risks is still largely absent within institutional environmental risk participatory mechanisms in all states that I explored (in the case of New York, public participants had to mobilize in unprecedented numbers to ensure a public health argument was included in HVHF deliberation). As the stasis analysis reveals, meaning-making about HVHF risk deliberation across states offers uneven access to deliberation tools about complex risk within HVHF practice. The routine lack of both precautionary and environmental justice ideologies within deliberation tools has potentially serious consequences in regards to both human and ecological health in regards to HVHF development. The next argument that I make is that activist literacy and invention patterns, informed by institutionally underrepresented ideologies of precaution and environmental justice, are compelling means of persuasion in representing environmental risk that enhance human and ecological health.

As difficult as these institutional mechanisms may be to navigate, my research shows that activist-driven representations of risk, invented *outside* of institutional reporting, have shown some success in advancing agency to influence some environmental risk assessment policy, a conclusion also found by Simmons and Grabill (2007). Counter-literacies can allow frames and ideologies to challenge "inevitable" HVHF activity as framed by dominant discourses (Dryzek, 2005). Intersectional precautionary and environmental justice frameworks found in New York's fracking ban, for example, challenge "industry" or "standard." But again, it is important to note that while these intersectional environmental justice frameworks might be feasible in some cases, the bulk of the language employed in policy tools offered to stakeholders suggests framing the environment simply as a resource. As such, very few institutional resources are offered to communities struggling with intersections of marginalization due to HVHF extraction.

The lack of precautionary or environmental justice frameworks in risk communication is a loss of an opportunity to create policies that account for the complex issues of environmental risk. Here I turn again to Royster and Kirsch (2012), this time to the feminist notion of strategic contemplation to encourage research that attends more clearly to complexities of environmental deliberation from public participants: "It allows scholars to observe and notice, to listen and hear voices often neglected and silenced (p. 85)." As such, I argue that HVHF activist voices are an important consideration in building better tools for HVHF deliberation.

The stasis analysis in this research reveals variations in deliberation possibilities based on definitions and jurisdictional policy decisions. CDA analysis in this research focuses on powerful policy choices that are informed by ideologies revealed in policy language. While the New York HVHF ban is important to explore, it is also crucial to understand that public participants who cannot access regulatory institutions that position human health concerns as an HVHF risk. These participants may not have the agency to offer technical knowledge if state or local laws do not "value" public health as an intersectional precautionary concern. Indeed, in Pennsylvania and Ohio, health officials have not been able to make a case to restrict HVHF activity based on health concerns. As stasis theory reveals, these are definitional ("IS"), value and jurisdictional ("OUGHT") concerns. There are other concerns about the deliberation of HVHF. In New York, activists are still positioned to do the work of "proving" the risk of HVHF infrastructure, transportation, storage, and disposal. Even highly technically literate public stakeholders might find that certain "sciences," "technologies" or types of expertise are not valued or even represented in risk reporting documents or processes (indeed, as energy risk assessment currently varies by state, state policies vary widely). My analysis of risk reporting tools reveals more deeply, the ways in which the power to "permit" HVHF activities is solidified and maintained through institutional mechanisms, resulting in a routine lack of procedural justice in terms of public access to defining and identifying HFHV risks and uncertainties in these states. Largely, legitimation of power in environmental discourse occurs through managerial approaches to permitting for industrial action. Additionally, there is reluctance to engage fully in energy options beyond extractive fossil fuels. These carbon fuels continue to have a hegemonic role in environmental policies in the United States.

This study examines only a small part of environmental risk reporting within larger studies of communication; however, it does attend to the socially situated nature of HVHF risk reporting. Past studies of environmental risk communication might include "psychometric methodologies" which explore how participants might use a particular tool without critical consideration of the tool in question. My study, which combines rhetorical analyses of contexts in which risk reporting tools might be used, and critical discourse analysis of language found within texts in risk reporting tools themselves, looks closely and critically at the tools participants are being asked to use. This combination of rhetorical and critical discourse analysis is unique to my study and informs ways in which citizens might engage in risk meaning-making to help to more clearly understand, as Grabill and Simmons suggest, ways in which literate tools might restrict citizens' roles in risk reporting (1998, p. 419).

My research answers calls for more situated research studies within rhetorics of science, public understandings of science, and rhetorics of risk and rhetorics informing technical and environmental communication. In response to the emergence of sustainability studies, several researchers call for rhetorics to promote public deliberation in the interest of a "sustainable future." These rhetorics might acknowledge possible deliberative spaces among varied authorities and ideological frameworks.

This study offers empirical data about these patterns that offer deeper understandings of environmental discourse analysis studies about energy and the environment with a concern about economic constructs, implicitly or explicitly referring to a "neoliberal" ideology. My research adds to the few existing legitimation scholarship projects about environmental discourse in that I explore participant responses as well as the institutional texts they must use (Steffek, 2009; Breeze, 2012). My primary data also augments studies about HVHF studies that explore how institutional contexts inform linguistic framing, and how those frames, in turn, might facilitate deliberations that explore transitions (or lack of transitions) in energy systems that move beyond carbon extraction: Stephens, Rand, and Melnick, 2009; Späth and Rohracher, 2010; Hoyt, 2012; Heikkila et al., 2014; Fuller and McCauley, 2016.

NOTES

1. Facing years of local public and legal opposition, plans from a private Texas industry to store forms of gas under Seneca Lake in New York were discontinued in 2017 (Murray, 2017).

2. As discussed in chapter 1, these environmental impact reports (which require public comment) are part of NEPA, or the National Environmental Policy Act of 1962, and are not required in all localities because HVHF is not yet defined, like coal mining, as an industry that might pose risk to the environment. Demonstration of "risk to the environment" must be made before an impact statement (and attendant public comment) is required.

3. This health study came about only after pressure was placed on the NY DEC to conduct such a study by public participants.

Chapter 5

Possibilities for Reframing Energy Discourse

Positive Discourse Analysis

In a 2022 *New York Times* article titled "There's a Messaging Battle Right Now Over America's Energy Future" authored by Gelles and Friedman, discuss how the term "energy transitions," brought about by the acknowledgment of rapid warming and change in the environment, has a different meaning depending on who is using it. For those in the oil and gas business, the transition is "a continued use of natural gas rather than coal" with a hoped-for carbon technology in the future; however, the authors note that this is still within the realm of fossil fuels. Other actors, mostly scientists, suggest the "rapid phasing out of fossil fuels and the immediate scaling up of cleaner energy sources like wind, solar, and nuclear." Gelles and Friedman point to Dr. Anthony Leiserowitz's work within language use at the Yale Program on Climate Change Communication, which acknowledges both greenwashing of terms like "transitions" and the opportunity for language that leads to new stories and new policies linked to truly renewable or sustainable energies that can help to mitigate the devastating effects of climate change. Renewable energy, sometimes also referred to as clean or green energy, is defined by the EIA (2022) to include biomass, hydropower, geothermal, wind, and solar energy supplies.

NEW YORK

Transitions are important to note as established in halting particular energy systems. Intersectional precautionary and environmental justice frameworks found in New York's fracking ban, for example, challenge "industry" or "standard." However, it is important to note that while these intersectional environmental justice frameworks might be feasible in some cases, the bulk of the language employed in policy tools offered to stakeholders suggests framing the environment simply as a resource linked to fossil fuel development. As such, very few institutional resources are offered to communities struggling with intersections of marginalization due to HVHF extraction or with imagining another type of future. As such, it is helpful to explore cases that consider energy transitions beyond fossil fuel expansion.

In this chapter, I explore how both positive and beneficial discourse analysis can be helpful in understanding how to effectively communicate energy transitions. Because of the advent of natural gas production, largely through fracking, fossil fuels continue to dominate energy production projections, despite climate change projections. As noted earlier in this book, the 2021 EIA (International Energy Information Administration) projects that worldwide natural gas is projected to increase by over 50 percent through the year 2050. While the EIA documents past growth and projects growth in the United States for renewable energy, renewable energy still only makes up 13.1 percent of U.S. primary energy consumption (2022). Also, the EIA cautions that projections depend upon "laws," "proposed legislation," and "regulations" (2022).

The Yale Program on Climate Change Communication is a rich source for leveraging climate change as a factor in discussions about energy transitions in the context of climate change. In addition to offering resources about climate change, it offers, to concerned citizens, explanations and links to research articles exploring energy transitions. For example, Olson-Hazboun, Howe, and Leiserowitz (2018) detail how public opinion on climate change and renewables depends on whether residents live near extractive activities (oil and gas production) and depends on political ideology. This can have social and cultural ramifications:

The politics of energy policy can thus become polarized among both political leaders and the general public based on ideological stances regarding the right of the government to "intervene" in the free market, for example by incentivizing one energy source over another through subsidies, as well as the decades old "jobs v. the environment" debate in which regulation of polluting energy sources is portrayed as an attack on blue-collar Americans (2018, p. 117).

Additionally, some may not view climate change as a threat or a short or long-term concern, depending on socio-spatial positionings.

The Yale Program on Climate Change Communication accesses information from the EIA to compare state renewable energy electricity production. According to their data, both Pennsylvania and Ohio produce on 3 percent of renewable energy for electric production. In New York, the number for renewable energy sources used for electricity production is 28 percent (Kirk, 2023). This brings about questions as to why adjacent states have such differing production rates, but also, how discursive practices might change in light of the pressing concerns of climate change.

Lucas et al.'s (2021) work on transforming public opinion about renewable energy reveals suggestions about communication strategies such as clear messaging in awareness campaigns and increasing public participation surrounding renewables. However, Duarte, Klarenbeek, Baetens, and Zegward (2016) discuss the importance of local vs. centrist or governmental initiatives in framing energy transitions. Dwortzan (2019) outlines a well-known MIT study that links Renewable Portfolio Standards (RPS), "which require electricity suppliers to source a designated percentage of electricity from available renewable-power generating technologies," to economic and human health benefits, particularly in the Rust Belt.

Positive and beneficial discourse analysis can be applied to renewable energy. What is most helpful here is the way these discourse patterns can frame new ways of discussing renewable energy. Arran Stibbe (2015) refers to Positive Discourse analysis as "the analysis of positive uses of language. i.e. ones which potentially help make the world a better place, as judged by the analyst's own ecosophy or values" (p. 205). In this case, ecological protection—including valuing the lives of species, including humans, is forefront. According to Stibbe (2005), this shifts the conversation from pointing out "oppressions and exploitations" to offering discourses "which are useful in facing contemporary challenges" (p. 31). While Stibbe cautions against romanticizing cultural sustainability language constructs, he offers an opportunity to explore language patterns that encourage deep sustainable change. In this case, he refers to ecosophy as being stories building what Jorgan Bang refers to as "ecological substantiality" or Larson's notion of "socio-ecological sustainability" (p. 11). These can include: how one values: living, well-being, the present and the future, environmental limits, social justice, and resilience.

Additionally, Stibbe (2015) refers to beneficial discourse analysis as "a discourse which conveys an ideology that accords with the ecosophy of the analyst (e.g., the discourse is seen as encouraging people to protect the ecosystem that life depends on)" (p. 201). These discourses link to earlier analysis, as revealed in the banning of HVHF drilling in New York, that have a theme of considering green storylines, intersectionality, and environmental justice.

Because, as noted before, New York has a much higher renewable electric production rate than the other states to which I was comparing, it is helpful to apply positive and beneficial discourse analysis to the renewables section of policies in New York. The New York State Energy Research and Development Authority—NYSERDA (founded in 1975) explores projections of renewable resources in the state. In this sense, it is not only important to show the potential ecological and human harms of HVHF, but also the opportunities of other energy systems. Many of the participants interviewed for this study noted their interest in supporting clean, green, or renewable energy. While it was outside the scope of data collection to gather TAPs of the renewable energy sites participants attended, it is important to note how institutions such as the NYSERDA offer positive and beneficial discourses.

As noted earlier in this book, Stibbe refers to language patterns that create "stories" with rich frames and embedded ideologies. Vocabulary, relationships between words, grammatical structures, assumptions and presuppositions, relationships between cause and effect, the way events and participants are represented, intertextuality, genres, and figures of speech all create a particular "story" (2015, p. 35).

On the NYSERDA site, "Clean Energy Standard" page, there is mention of "leadership" in the Climate Leadership and Community Protection Act in the state of New York, which has a goal of "generating 70% of our power from renewables by 2030." First, this positions New York as a state actor striving toward a future of protecting citizens, in part, through renewable energy policy.

The site offers practical links for residents to access large- and small-scale renewable energy projects, including solar, hydro, and wind projects. Throughout the site, there is mention of responding to climate change, finding low-carbon alternatives, and a renewable energy infrastructure. But there is also a link to financial incentives offered through the state: "Investment in New York's renewable energy transition can be seen through more than $29 billion in public and private investment which includes nearly 100 onshore solar, wind and hydro, and offshore wind projects; as well as investments in transmission as part of constructing New York's Green Energy Transmission Superhighway" (2023), linking to an economic ideology. The site details credits for renewable energy and zero emissions and future projects, such as offshore wind initiatives and revitalization projects "prioritizing the development of existing or abandoned commercial sites, brownfields, landfills, former industrial sites, and other abandoned or underutilized sites." (2023). Here, the relationship from a past carbon economy is shifted to new possibilities of a green economy. The story that emerges, linguistically from this site, is that renewables can offer a triple win of economic, environmental, and community health.

Additionally, the site offers resources for local governments to encourage renewable energy projects—all linking to the assumption of a future where renewables would be embraced. Unlike the permitting for fracking so often seen on Ohio and Pennsylvania's institutional pages, the Clean Energy Siting Resources page offers practical and technical assistance to site renewable energy in local communities. The terms "empower" and "implementation of clean energy" offer an alternative storyline to the assumption about the public embracing natural gas in Ohio and Pennsylvania. The site reveals an assumption of the awareness of climate change and practical strategies to embrace a future that might attend to the radical lowering of carbon emissions. Perhaps what is most compelling about this small sampling within this site is the storyline of an ecology that is being protected through socially constructed green energy infrastructure.

OHIO AND PENNSYLVANIA

Positive discourse analysis supporting alternative energy infrastructure can also be seen in both Ohio and Pennsylvania, but successful narratives about post-carbon futures often link to past work practices. While opportunities in both Ohio and Pennsylvania for post-carbon economies are not as prevalent as in New York, there are stories of participants engaging in alternatives to HVHF.

For example, the group ReImagine Appalachia, which serves both Ohio and Pennsylvania in the Ohio River Valley, digs into rust belt and Appalachian ideologies to call for a holistic grassroots effort to address transitions from extractive economies in rust belt and Appalachian spaces. Resources include blueprints for building communities and workspaces that link to a sustainable economy.

By honoring and fore fronting the work ethic of past steel, mining, and industrial spaces, this nonprofit group, which brings coalitions of other nonprofits together, and is able to trace a powerful story that retains the original character of workers from an extractive economy while suggesting a post-carbon economy. ReImagine Appalachia invites plans and offers links to grants for a post-carbon economy by focusing on the storyline of dignity of long-term sustainable work. This group explores sustainable city "hubs" that would offer climate resiliency in the Ohio River Valley. The group focuses on green manufacturing (in the wind, solar, and geothermal sectors), as well as calls for long-term jobs for remediating lands that have suffered from past extractions, such as orphan well, methane reduction, and mining remediation efforts. Additionally, the storyline within this group discusses how a Climate Corps (reminiscent of the Civilian Conservation Corps) can open up work opportunities in Appalachia.

This group is interesting because it uses a well-known storyline: "work"—but transitions the discussion from past extractive economies to long-term and inclusive workspaces, and includes a discussion of mutual well-being (earth and humans):

> In response, a diverse set of economic, environmental and community leaders, and grassroots organizations, came together to find common ground and build

> the future we want to see—a 21st century economy that's good for workers, communities, and the environment.

While the discussion is rooted in economic wealth, the turn is toward "local" wealth, and resources often discuss holistic opportunities in towns that had once seen short-term wealth based on extractive economies:

> Today we stand united, building on the power of past efforts to define our own future—one grounded in our land and centered on creating local wealth. We need both a vision and a plan. Both must rely on our skilled workers and farmers while also offering hope for our next generation—of all races, ethnicities, and genders. (ReImagine Appalachia, 2024)

ReImagine Appalachia continues a narrative of reimagined work by offering detailed community benefits plans, including legal and grant writing capabilities, links to grassroots organizations, and working case studies. These case studies reveal successful solar and other alternative energy infrastructure in a variety of cities, offering a glimpse of what could "be" beyond extractive economies so prevalent in the past, while not rejecting that past outright.

Conclusion

This research reveals socially situated constraints and affordances surrounding literacies that activist participants navigate in an effort to tell stories about environmental risk as related to the HVHF industry. The stories told by activists offer opportunities to name risk in existing HVHF activity and offer alternative considerations for energy development. It is worthy to note how important "place" is in the studying regions—the rust belt and Appalachian regions often accept HVHF as inevitable, but nearby states (New York) are able to stop HVHF build-out by using an environmental lens.

When activists were stymied in deliberation while using institutional environmental risk participatory mechanisms, they turned to various counter-literacies to tell nuanced stories of HVHF environmental risk; in the case of New York, these counter-literacies expanded notions of HVHF risk and impacted New York environmental policy in terms of the HVHF drilling ban. I make two arguments based on my data. One is that public access to meaningful deliberation about HVHF environmental risks is still largely absent within institutional environmental risk participatory mechanisms in all states that I explored (in the case of New York, public participants had to mobilize in unprecedented numbers to ensure a public health argument was included in HVHF deliberation). As the stasis analysis reveals, meaning-making about HVHF risk deliberation across states offers uneven access to deliberation tools about complex risk within HVHF practice. Where you live impacts how you can tell a story about a place. The routine lack of both precautionary and environmental justice ideologies within deliberation tools has potentially serious consequences in regard to both human and ecological health in regards to HVHF development. The next argument that I make is that activist literacy and invention patterns, informed by institutionally underrepresented ideologies of precaution and environmental justice, are compelling means of persuasion in representing environmental risk that enhance human and ecological health, as is revealed in the positive and beneficial discourses found in New York's institutional sites paving the path for renewable energy.

As difficult as these institutional mechanisms may be to navigate, my research shows that activist-driven representations of risk invented *outside* of institutional reporting have shown some success in advancing agency to influence some environmental risk assessment policy, a conclusion also found by Simmons and Grabill (2007). Counter-literacies can allow frames and ideologies to challenge "inevitable" HVHF activity as framed by dominant discourses (Dryzek, 2005). In New York, what has become "inevitable," through a positive and beneficial discourse lens, is renewable energy.

The lack of precautionary or environmental justice frameworks in risk communication in other states is a loss of an opportunity to create policies that account for complex issues of environmental risk. Here, I turn again to Royster and Kirsch (2012), this time to the feminist notion of strategic contemplation to encourage research that attends more clearly to the complexities of environmental deliberation from public participants: "It allows scholars to observe and notice, to listen and hear voices often neglected and silenced (p. 85)." As such, I argue that HVHF activist voices are an important consideration in building better tools for HVHF deliberation.

The stasis analysis in this research reveals variations in deliberation possibilities based on definitions and jurisdictional policy decisions. CDA analysis in this research focuses on powerful policy choices that are informed by ideologies revealed in policy language. While the New York HVHF ban is important to explore, it is also crucial to understand that public participants who cannot access regulatory institutions that position human health concerns as an HVHF risk. These participants may not have the agency to offer technical knowledge if state or local laws do not "value" public health as an intersectional precautionary concern. Indeed, in Pennsylvania and Ohio, health officials have not been able to make a case to restrict HVHF activity based on health concerns. As stasis theory reveals, these are definitional ("IS"), value, and jurisdictional ("OUGHT") concerns. There are other concerns about the deliberation of HVHF. In New York, activists are still positioned to do the work of "proving" risk of HVHF infrastructure, transportation, storage, and disposal, even as renewables are embraced. Even highly technically literate public stakeholders might find that certain "sciences," "technologies," or types of expertise are not valued or even represented in risk reporting documents or processes (indeed, as energy risk assessment currently varies by state, state policies vary widely). My analysis of risk reporting tools reveals more deeply the ways in which the power to "permit" for HVHF activities is solidified and maintained through institutional mechanisms, resulting in a routine lack of procedural justice in terms of public access to defining and identifying HVHF risks and uncertainties in states like Ohio and Pennsylvania. Largely, the legitimation of power in environmental discourse occurs through managerial approaches to permitting for industrial action. Additionally, there is reluctance to engage fully in energy options beyond the extractive fossil fuels. These carbon fuels continue to have a hegemonic role in environmental policies in the United States. However, by looking at activist work, one can see how spaces like Pennsylvania and Ohio can tap into ideologies to enable participation in more meaningful ways.

This study examines only a small part of environmental risk reporting within larger studies of communication; however, it does attend to the socially situated nature of HVHF risk reporting. Past studies of environmental risk communication might include "psychometric methodologies" which explore how participants might use a particular tool without critical consideration of the tool in question. My study, which combines rhetorical analyses of contexts in which risk reporting tools might be used, and critical discourse analysis of language found within texts in risk reporting tools themselves, looks closely and critically at the tools participants are being asked to use. This combination of rhetorical and critical discourse analysis is unique to my study and informs ways in which citizens might engage in risk meaning-making to help to more clearly understand, as Grabill and Simmons suggest, ways in which literate tools might to restrict citizens' roles in risk reporting (1998, p. 419).

My research answers calls for more situated research studies within rhetorics of science, public understandings of science, and rhetorics of risk and rhetorics informing technical and environmental communication—particularly as linked to "place." In response to the emergence of sustainability studies, several researchers call for rhetorics to promote public deliberation in the interest of a "sustainable future." These studies should be informed by community groups that are intimately aware of the ideologies of a particular place. These rhetorics might acknowledge possible deliberative spaces among varied authorities and ideological frameworks.

This study offers empirical data about these patterns that offer deeper understandings of environmental discourse analysis studies about energy and the environment with a concern about economic constructs, implicitly or explicitly referring to a "neoliberal" ideology. My research adds to the few existing legitimation scholarship projects about environmental discourse in that I explore participant responses as well as the institutional texts they must use (Steffek, 2009; Breeze, 2012). My primary data also augment studies about HVHF studies that explore how institutional contexts inform linguistic framing, and how those frames, in turn, might facilitate deliberations that explore transitions (or lack of transitions) in energy systems that move beyond carbon extraction: Stephens, Rand, and Melnick, 2009; Späth and

Rohracher, 2010; Hoyt, 2012; Heikkila et al., 2014; Fuller and McCauley, 2016.

In addition to rhetorical and CDA contextual and textual analysis, my research explores ways individuals make meaning about environmental risk. This aspect informs literacy studies that explore community literacies. In particular, there are very few literacy studies that look closely at the risk reporting tools used by participants to assess environmental risk, particularly in situated spaces. Even fewer have explored participants' use of technical literacy tools as they navigate environmental risk issues to make meaning outside of institutional constructs. My focus on invention as practiced within community literacies offers primary data to more fully understand the call for varied authorities to make meaning about environmental risk (Goggin, 2009; Buizer, Arts, and Kok, 2011; Scholz, 2011; Herndl and Cutlip, 2013). My work also informs language scholarship that focuses more specifically on risk, science, and stakeholders.

Increasingly, calls for research within technical and environmental communication scholarship emphasizes the importance of focusing on communication among various stakeholders, local knowledges, and participatory methods in these conversations, as well as evaluations of those public participation methods in environmental issues. My work offers analysis to further understand the ways in which participatory methods can be improved, in particular, by offering analysis of primary data about intersectionality, precaution, and environmental justice. My work also intersects with scholarship about environmental communication that explores how technical science is communicated to and by public participants, providing empirical data to scholarship that showcases the possibilities of praxis within technical communication: Carolan, 2008; Klein, 2010; Condit, 2012; Ceccerali, 2013; Druschke and Gottschalk, 2014.

This research also speaks to scholarship in fields that explore links between the environment and public health, energy policy, energy production, and risk (including research calls from institutional agencies, such as the EPA). As suggested earlier, this research attends to emerging calls from fields such as sustainability sciences or fields exploring notions of sustainability to situate research about communication surrounding complex environmental-social issues. In particular, several fields are calling for studies of intersectional and feminist approaches (both theoretical and empirical studies) to better address complex environmental issues. There are considerable questions as to how notions of complex "intersectionality" might be part of public policy deliberations, specifically about existing and emerging energy extraction systems such as HVHF. Scholarship in geography and environmental studies suggest gaps between ideological frames of different groups deliberating about HVHF policy. Federal, state, and local leaders often have the agency to support and implement HVHF extraction systems by making short-term economic arguments for the industry; as such, the industry often becomes "institutionalized" before meaningful public deliberation. By contrast, publics who will live with and near HVHF extraction, production, and transport sites may point to a variety of social, economic, and health concerns that may be compounded through time (Beinkowski, 2015). These public participants, however, may not have the agency or opportunity to publicly articulate such complex concerns (Heikkila et al., 2014; Crowe, Silva, Ceresola, Buday, and Leonard, 2015; Isreal, Wong-Parodi, Webler, and Stern, 2015; Dignum et al., 2016; Kinchy, Parks, and Jalbert, 2016). Such gaps may lead to "citizen science" initiatives (Kinchy, Parks, and Jalbert, 2016), or citizen-based deliberations about HFHV. But, it is currently acknowledged that these wider, intersecting definitions of HVHF risk are not found in "expert-led" deliberations (Isreal et al., 2015, p. 139). My study specifically offers discursive analysis about many intersectional concerns within geography and environmental studies scholarship interrogating HVHF risk.

This study adds to the understanding how procedural justice in terms of accessing relevant information to represent environmental risks, particularly in terms of emerging technologies, might be highlighted within broader environmental risk assessment communication. This comparative research also enters into discussions about global environmental deliberation, particularly in light of socially constructed policies that address risks that do not stay fixed in space. I center my study on HVHF risk in three states, but this small study offers empirical research about deliberative capacity to confront complex environmental issues across political borders. For example, Dryzek (2013) largely notes the constraints of current political deliberative capacity to enact policy about climate change. Dryzek defines deliberative capacity as "the degree to which a system hosts authentic, inclusive, and consequential deliberation." Instead of current adversarial democracy models, he suggests the possibilities of more deliberative, consensual democracies (2013). While my study does not look at global climate change, the subject of Dryzek's theory of deliberative democracy, it provides empirical evidence in terms of activists participating in deliberative democracies to shape local policy in regard to HVHF risk representation that links to wider discussions about energy systems and, as in the case of New York, changes in policy. It is hoped that the research offered in this book, in conjunction with other empirical research, offers some tools, particularly in light of precautionary discourses, to environmental risk assessment and deliberation about complex and uncertain risks.

LIMITATIONS AND FUTURE STUDY POSSIBILITIES

My research certainly has its limitations in terms of Dryzek's suggestion of understanding consensual democratic deliberation and subsequent policy performance.

My research is centered only on three states from a general geographical area in the United States (the Rust Belt) and included only eighteen participants who all identified as activists. My participants were all similar in terms of race and class. As such, there are many other geographical "identities" and other populations that might reveal further understanding of deliberative possibility about HVHF (including international approaches) to more clearly understand environmental justice concerns in terms of race (Bullard, 1993) and class (Nixon, 2011). As noted in chapter 1, this study looks at only a small part of environmental risk reporting within larger studies of environmental risk communication; however, it does attend to the socially situated nature of this risk reporting.

As a study based on empirical research methods, this study might contribute to other emerging studies that consider multi-modality in environmental risk assessment usability. This study offers one of the few studies within environmental communication that highlights participant navigation through multimodal texts. Given the scope of my research, I was not able to fully analyze multimodal visuals or semiotics that might represent risks (or, in some cases, obscure risks) within tools that participants might navigate or create. This notion of multi-modality within technical environmental deliberation is particularly salient and is a possible future study possibility within existing data. Dobrin and Morey's *EcoSee: Image, Rhetoric, Nature* (2009) offers helpful frameworks for visual analysis that would be useful for the visual data in this study. Tim Bowers' (2005) work explores the rhetorical implications of visual images that depict environmental justice concerns, which also might be applied to my data collection. Research in CDA includes analysis frames for multimodal discourses (Kress, 2012) and multimedia discourses (Kress, 2012). These studies offer rich possibilities for this project in terms of future studies based on participant navigation and suggest additional questions about online public spaces and questions about how issues of power are framed within text navigation itself.

Additionally, I hinted at "precautionary" discourses, but, given the scope of my study, suggest that a rich area of inquiry is to look into participants' concerns about environmental risks over time. All participants voiced concern about environmental degradation over time. Rob Nixon frames this kind of environmental concern as "slow" environmental violence, which theorizes that environmental risk compounds with intersecting risks through time, a concern that might be explored in more detail (2011). Harré, Brockmeier, and Mühlhäusler's (1999) constructions of language and time as related to environmental processes are an important consideration in risk representation that I was not able to include in this dissertation and offer considerations for future study. Additional questions about time might include ways in which institutions plan for and represent environmental degradation over time. Additionally, most institutional sites discuss "restoration" of an HVHF activity site while simultaneously claiming HVHF activity is causing no harm. A deeper investigation into the notion of HVHF "restoration" is a future research possibility.

As noted in chapter 1, it is important to continue to interrogate *why* "counter-public discourse" storytelling and participation possibilities are routinely not included as part of environmental risk assessments, which are regularly marked by issues of procedural justice related to institutional literacies in terms of representing environmental risk. In sum, my research is an attempt to bring to the forefront moments where activists invent beyond these "objective" technical models to consider ways in which a larger deliberation about environmental risk might occur, particularly in times where global environmental issues are increasingly a concern, and how to communicate and create praxis about these concerns. This expanded notion of environmental risk assessment is an increasingly pressing matter in a world dealing with long-term environmental concerns such as global climate change and its attendant complexities.

Appendices

APPENDIX A: INTERVIEW QUESTIONS

The research session, which includes interviews and observations, can take up to *approximately three hours to three and a half hours on one day*. Some participants may be invited to participate in a follow-up interview. A follow-up interview is optional and will take *approximately one to two hours* on another date. All procedures will take place in a public setting or private setting, mutually agreed upon by the participants and the co-investigator.[1] A participant can opt out at any time.

Interviews and Observations (*Three to three and a half hours in one day*)

Project participants will be asked to participate in an interview about the reading and writing used to navigate local, state, and federal environmental risk sites and documents. This interview should take about 30–45 minutes.

In addition, participants will be asked to participate in an observation (this is called a think-aloud protocol) in which the co-investigator will ask participants to recount their thought process aloud as they read through local, state, and federal environmental risk sites or documents. This observation should take about 45 minutes to one hour.

Participants will next be asked to participate in an interview about the reading and writing used to navigate sites or documents *outside* of local, state, and federal environmental risk sites and documents to understand environmental risks. This could include participants' own writing or writing they have collaborated on with others. This interview should take about 30–45 minutes.

Finally, in the last observation, the co-investigator will ask participants to recount their thought process aloud as they read through documents *outside* of local, state, and federal risk sites and documents. This could include their own writing or writing they have collaborated on with others. These could be publicly shared documents such as meeting handouts, blogs, Facebook posts, published scholarly research, and newspaper editorials and news sites. Each observation should take about 45 minutes to one hour.

Some participants may be asked for follow-up interviews (one to two hours). Should participants be asked, this interview is optional. These will take place on a separate day. Again, these interviews will take place in a public or private mutually agreed upon location between the participant and co-investigator.

Interview Questions, Set 1: Reporting Risks within Local, State and Federal Risk Reporting Sites (*30–45 Minutes*)

Co-Investigator: Thank you for participating. I will be asking you questions about how you read and write about environmental risks. I want to remind you that answering any of these questions is voluntary. If we would like to speak further about questions I ask today, I will e-mail you and set up another interview, but only if you agree. All interviews are voluntary. The first set of interview questions will discuss how you have tried to learn about or report environmental risks using local, state or federal sites or procedures. After we talk about these, if you have reported or learned about environmental risks in spaces besides local, state or federal sites or procedures, I will ask questions about them. Are you ready to begin?

1. What is your definition of an environmental risk? Feel free to talk about examples from your own life.
2. What is your understanding of how you can report an environmental risk?
3. What local internet sites/reporting documents have you used to understand or report environmental risk concerns?
4. What aspects of environmental risk reporting, using these local internet sites/reporting documents, have you found to be effective? Why?
    a. For example, was the language in readings approachable? Why or why not?
    b. Were you able to respond to written requests? Why or why not?
    c. Were time frames for reporting various risks reasonable? Why or why not?

5. What aspects of environmental risk reporting, using these local internet sites/reporting documents, have you found to be problematic? Why?
   a. For example, was the language in readings not approachable? Why or why not?
   b. Were you not able to respond to written requests? Why or why not?
   c. Were time frames for reporting various risks not reasonable? Why or why not?
6. What state internet sites/reporting documents have you used to understand or report environmental risk concerns?
7. What aspects of environmental risk reporting, using these state internet sites/reporting documents, have you found to be effective? Why?
   a. For example, was the language in readings approachable? Why or why not?
   b. Were you able to respond to written requests? Why or why not?
   c. Were time frames for reporting various risks reasonable? Why or why not?
8. What aspects of environmental risk reporting, using these state internet sites/reporting documents, have you found to be problematic? Why?
   a. For example, was the language in readings approachable? Why or why not?
   b. Were you able to respond to written requests? Why or why not?
   c. Were time frames for reporting various risks reasonable? Why or why not?
9. What federal internet sites/reporting documents have you used to understand or report environmental risk concerns?
10. What aspects of environmental risk reporting, using these federal internet sites/reporting documents, have you found to be effective. Why?
    a. For example, was the language in readings approachable? Why or why not?
    b. Were you able to respond to written requests? Why or why not?
    c. Were time frames for reporting various risks reasonable? Why or why not?
11. What aspects of environmental risk reporting, using these federal internet sites/reporting documents, have you found to be problematic? Why?
    a. For example, was the language in readings approachable? Why or why not?
    b. Were you able to respond to written requests? Why or why not?
    c. Were time frames for reporting various risks reasonable? Why or why not?

APPENDIX B

Tap

Think-Aloud Protocol 1 *(45 minutes to 1 hour)*

The co-investigator will read the following:

I will be observing you as you think your thoughts aloud. This lets me understand, at least in part, the thought process you have as you use a product, device, or manual or complete a task, like writing. I'll observe you while the you attempt to complete a defined task. Ideally, I'll only speaks to remind you to "please keep talking."

By thinking aloud while attempting to complete the task, you can explain their method of attempting to complete the task, and illuminate any difficulties you encounter in the process. Here, I will be asking you to consider ways in which you encounter issues, and problem solve when reading and writing about environmental risks.

Before we begin that, we will practice the think aloud process. As noted on the consent form, I will be audio taping your responses.

For practice, please think aloud to count up the number of windows in your parent's home. Please try to think this problem out loud, so try to include any details in the task. Try to say everything aloud that leads up to you solving this problem.

If you feel uncomfortable, you may stop at any time. If you have a question about the task, you may ask, but I will not be able to answer. I may prompt you to continue talking. You will determine the end of the task. When you feel you have completed the task, please let me know.

After this stage, the co-investigator will read the following:

Now we will apply the think aloud to texts you have gathered for the way you read and write about environmental risk. Please discuss aloud how you move through the sites we discussed in the interview to understand environmental risk. Discuss aloud the ways these sites present environmental risks—how you would use or have used these sites is fine. Feel free to spend time on any part of the site (we will finish at the approximate end of an hour). If you feel uncomfortable, you may stop at any time. I may prompt you to continue talking. You will determine the end of the task. When you feel you have completed the task, please let me know. Do you have any questions before we begin?

Interview Questions, Set 2 (*30–45 minutes*)

Co-Investigator: I will now ask you questions about how you read and write about environmental risks outside of local, state, and federal risk reporting sites or procedures. I want to remind you that answering any of these questions is voluntary. If we would like to speak further about questions I ask today, I will e-mail you and set up another interview, but only if you agree. All interviews are voluntary. This time, I would like to talk to you about reading and writing you do about environmental risks that might not be sponsored by local, state or federal regulations. Are you ready to begin?

1. In what ways have you found alternative ways to report or alert communities about environmental risk concerns? Feel free to think about any way you read or write about environmental risks. Is this a concern that you feel is something you can report to a governmental institution?
   a. If yes, can you describe the reading and writing you did to understand or report this risk?
   b. If no, how were you first alerted that this was a concern not covered by existing environmental risk reporting?
2. How did you research the issue? Can you give specifics about websites, scholarly articles, community groups, research techniques etc. that helped you to research?
3. Did you have any difficulty reading through any of the material? Why or Why not?
   a. If yes, what did you do when you had difficulty reading material?
4. Did you have any difficulty in writing about this issue? Why or Why not?
   a. If yes, what did you do when you had difficulty writing about this issue?
5. How did you organize your findings? What led you to arrange your findings in the way in which you did?
6. Did you collaborate with any groups to share your findings? How?
7. Did you feel that you could share your findings about environmental risk in your community in spaces that would address your concerns? Why or why not?
8. If you are reporting risks that aren't covered by local, state and federal reporting, why do you think the environmental risk concerns that you are exploring are not part of institutional local, state or federal risk reporting?

9. In response to the last question, do you think that these concerns will be part of later institutional risk assessments?

Think-Aloud Protocol 2 (*45 min–1 hour*)

The co-investigator will read the following:

I will be observing you as you think your thoughts aloud. This lets me understand, at least in part, the thought process you have as you use a product, device, or manual or complete a task, like writing. I'll observe you while the you attempt to complete a defined task. Ideally, I'll only speaks to remind you to "please keep talking."

By thinking aloud while attempting to complete the task, you can explain their method of attempting to complete the task, and illuminate any difficulties you encounter in the process. Here, I will be asking you to consider ways in which you encounter issues, and problem solve when reading and writing about environmental risks.

After this stage, the co-investigator will read the following:

Now we will apply the think aloud to the way you read and write about environmental risk outside of the risk reporting sites we explored earlier. Please discuss aloud how you read or composed documents to explore environmental risk outside of the sites we went over during the first observation. This discussion could be about any form you have created or others have created: digital or paper is fine. Feel free to spend time on any part of the reading or writing you have done to report risk. We will finish approximately at the end of the hour. If you feel uncomfortable, you may stop at any time. I may prompt you to continue talking. You will determine the end of the task. When you feel you have completed the task, please let me know. Do you have any questions before we begin?

APPENDIX C

Local, State, and Federal Risk Reporting Agencies

Ohio	Ohio Department of Natural **Resources** • State: http://oilandgas.ohiodnr.gov/ • Ohio EPA (Environmental Protection Agency): state group does not work with public comment for unconventional gas activities sent back to ODNR http://www.epa.state.oh.us/ • Local: • OH LEPC & SERC (local and state hazardous material reporting)
Pennsylvania	Pennsylvania Department of **Conservatio**n and Natural **Resources** • State: http://www.dcnr.state.pa.us/forestry/NaturalGas/index.htm (state game lands, not private lands) • Department of Environmental **Protection**: http://www.depweb.state.pa.us/portal/server.pt/community/dep_home/5968 • County: http://www.co.greene.pa.us/secured/gc2/government.htm • PA LEPC & SERC (local and state hazardous material reporting)
New York	New York State Department of Natural **Conservation** • State:http://www.dec.ny.gov/60.html • New York State Department of Health: https://www.health.ny.gov/ • Township (Dryden):http://dryden.ny.us/information/gas-drilling-info
Federal	• U.S. Department of Energy: http://www.energy.gov/eere/energybasics/articles/glossary-energy-related-terms • EPA (federal): http://www.epa.gov/ • Federal Energy Regulatory Commission: http://www.ferc.gov/

NOTE

1. Federal IRB (institutional review board) regulations require an advisor to be listed as the "Primary Investigator" and a graduate researcher to be listed as the "Co-Investigator."

References

Abandoned Mine Reclamation Clearinghouse. n.d. "SMCRA Surface Mining Control and Reclamation Act of 1977 and the Abandoned Mine Reclamation Fund". http://www.amrclearinghouse.org/Sub/LEGAL/SMCRA.htm.

Adler, Jonathan. 2004. "The Fable of Environmental Regulation: Reconsidering the Federal Role in Environmental Protection." *Case Western Law Review,* 55(1), 93–113.

Alaimo, Stacy. 2008. "Trans-Corporeal Feminisms and the Ethical Space of Nature." In *Material Feminisms,* edited by Stacy Alaimo & Susan Hekman, 236–250. Bloomington: Indiana University Press.

Bäckstrand, Karen. 2003. "Civic Science for Sustainability: Reframing the Role of Experts, Policy-Makers and Citizens in Environmental Governance." *Global Environmental Ethics,* 3(4), 24–41.

Beck, Ulrich. 1987. "Risk Society and the Provident State." In *Risk, Environment, & Modernity: Towards a New Ecology*, edited by Scott Lash, Bronislaw Szerszynski, & Brian Wynne, 27–43. London: Sage.

Bienkowski, Brian. 2015. "Poor in Pennsylvania? You're Fracked." *Environmental Health News,* May 6, 2016, http://www.environmentalhealthnews.org/ehs/news/2015/may/pennsylvania-fracking-environmental-justice-pooreconomics.

Black, Brian, & Ladson, M. 2012. "The Legacy of Extraction: Reading Patterns and Ethics in Pennsylvania's Landscape of Energy." *Environmental Histories of the Mid-Atlantic,* 79(4), 377–394.

Blommaert, Jan. 2003. "A Sociolinguistics of Globalization." *Journal of Sociolinguistics,* 7(4), 433–448.

Blommaert, Jan, & Bulcaen, C. 2000. "Critical Discourse Analysis." *Annual Review of Anthropology,* 29, 447–466.

Blythe, Stuart, Grabill, J., & Riley, K. (2008). "Action Research and Wicked Environmental Problems: Exploring Appropriate Roles for Researchers in Professional Communication." *Journal of Business and Technical Communication,* 22(3), 272–299.

Bowers, Tom. 2005. *Rationality and Environmental Justice: The Visual Rhetoric of a Culture at Risk* (Doctoral dissertation). Iowa State University Digital Repository.

Brady, W. 2011. *Hydraulic Fracturing Regulation in the United States: The Laissez-Faire Approach of the Federal Government and Varying State Regulations.* Denver, CO: University of Denver, Sturm College of Law.

Breeze, Ruth. 2012. "Legitimation in Corporate Discourse: Oil Corporations after Deepwater Horizon." *Discourse & Society,* 23(1), 3–18.

Brulle, Robert. 2010. "Politics and the Environment." In *The Handbook of Politics: State and Civil Society in Global Perspective,* edited by Kevin T. Leicht & J. Craig Jenkins, 385–406. New York: Springer Publishers.

Buizer, Marteen, Arts, B., and Kok, K. 2011. "Governance, Scale, and the Environment: the Importance of Recognizing Knowledge Claims in Transdisciplinary Arenas." *Ecology and Society* 16(1), 21.

Bullard, Robert. 1993. "Race and Environmental Justice in the United States." *Yale Journal of International Law,* 18(1), 319–335.

"Business and Industry." n.d. *Ohio History Central.* Accessed 2017, http://www.ohiohistorycentral.org/w/Category:Business_and_Industry.

Cantrill, Jame. 1996. "Gold, Yellowstone and the Search for a Rhetorical Identity." In *Green Culture: Environmental Rhetoric in Contemporary America,* 166–194. Madison: University of Wisconsin Press.

Carolan, Michael. 2008. "The Bright and Blind Spots of Science: Why Objective Knowledge is not Enough to Resolve Environmental Controversies." *Critical Sociologies,* 34(7), 725–740.

Ceccarelli, Leah. 2013. "To Whom do We Speak? The Audiences for Scholarship on the Rhetoric of Science and Technology. *Poroi,* 9, 1.

Center for Coalfield Justice. n.d. "What we Do." https://www.coalfieldjustice.org/what-we-do.

Center for Coalfield Justice. 2013. "Community Indicators of Environmental Justice: A Baseline Report Focusing on Greene and Washington Counties, Pennsylvania." Colcom Foundation.

Center for Health, Environment & Justice, Ohio. n.d. http://66.39.116.85/ohio.htm.

Chesapeake Bay Foundation. n.d. Natural Gas Drilling. http://www.cbf.org/issues/natural-gas-drilling/index.html.

Chesapeake Bay Foundation. n.d. Pollution limits by state. http://www.cbf.org/how-we-save-the-bay/chesapeake-clean-water-blueprint/pollution-limits/pollution-limits-by-state.html?referrer=https://www.google.com/.

Comfort, Susan. 2017. "Rusted Futures: Uneven Development, Activist stories, and Ecofeminist Challenges in Northern Appalachia's Coal Country." Lecture session presented at the meeting of the Association for the Study of Literature and Environment, Detroit, MI.

Condit, Celeste, Lynch, J., & Winderman, E. 2012. "Recent Rhetorical Studies in Public Understanding of Science: Multiple Purposes and Strengths. *Public Understanding of Science,* 21(4), 386–400.

Conrad, Cathy, & Hilchey, K. 2011. A Review of Citizen Science and Community-based Environmental Monitoring: Issues and Opportunities. *Environmental Monitoring and Assessment*, 176(1–4), 273–291.

Cox, Robert. 2006. *Environmental Communication and the Public Sphere*. Thousand Oaks, CA: Sage.

Crowe, Jessica, Silva, T., Ceresola, R., Buday, A., & Leonard, C. 2015. "Differences in PublicPerceptions and Leaders' Perceptions on Hydraulic Fracturing and Shale Development." *Sociological Perspectives,* 58(3), 441–463.

Curran, Glorel. 2012. "Contested Energy Futures: Shaping Renewable Energy Narratives in Australia." *Global Climate Change*, 22(1), 236–244.

Cutcliffe, Stephen. 2012. "From Seed Men to Bird Women: Pennsylvanians and the Environment." *Pennsylvania History: A Journal of Mid-Atlantic Studies,* 79(4), 495–506.

Davies, Kate. 2013. *The Rise of the Environmental Health Movement.* Lanham, MD: Rowman and Littlefield.

Dietz, Thomas, & Stern, Paul C. (Eds.). 2008. *Public Participation in Environmental Assessment and Decision Making.* Washington D.C.: The National Academies Press.

Dignum, Marloes, Correlje, A., Cuppen, E., Pesch, U., & Taebi, B. 2016. "Contested Technologies and Design for Values: The Case of Shale Gas." *Science and Engineering Ethics*, 22(1), 1171–1191.

Dobrin, Sidney, & Morey, S. (Eds.). 2009. *Ecosee: Image, Rhetoric, Nature.* New York: State University of New York Press.

Druschke, Caroline G. 2014. "With Whom do We Speak? Building Transdisciplinary Collaborations in the Rhetoric of Science." *Poroi,* 10(1), 1–7.

Dryzek, John S. 2005. *The Politics of the Earth: Environmental Discourses*. Oxford: Oxford University Press.

Dryzek, John S. 2013. *Center for Humans and Nature.* Retrieved from http://www.humansandnature.org/democracy-john-dryzek.

Duarte, F., Klarenbeek, L., Baetens, J., & Zegwaard, A. 2016. "Do it yourself, Together: A Discourse Analysis on How People Talk about Local Initiatives for Renewable Energy." *Communication, Behavior & Sustainable Society,* 1–16. https://research.hanze.nl/en/publications/do-it-yourself-together-a-discourse-analysis-on-how-people-talk-a.

Dwortzan. Mark. 2019. "Shift to Renewable Electricity a Win-win at Statewide Level." *MIT.* https://news.mit.edu/2019/shift-renewable-electricity-win-win-statewide-level-0814.

"Early Industrialization, Ohio." n.d. *Ohio History Central.* http://www.ohiohistorycentral.org/w/Early_Industrialization.

Easterling, D. R., & Karl, T. R. 2001. "Potential Consequences of Climate Variability and Change for the Midwestern United States". In *Climate Change Impacts on the United States: The Potential Consequences of Climate Variability and Change.* National Assessment Team, U.S. Global Change Research Program.

Edmonson, B. 2001. "Environmental Affairs in New York State: An Historical Overview." *New York State Archives*, 72.

Energy Information Administration. 2015. "Fossil Fuels Still Dominate U.S. Energy Consumption." https://www.eia.gov/todayinenergy/detail.php?id=26912.

Energy Information Administration. 2021a. "How Much of U.S. Energy." https://www.eia.gov/tools/faqs/faq.php?id=92&t=4.

Energy Information Administration. 2021b. "International." https://www.eia.gov/international/overview/world.

Energy Information Administration. 2021c. "Natural Gas Explained." https://www.eia.gov/energyexplained/natural-gas/where-our-natural-gas-comes-from.php.

Energy Information Administration. 2021d. "Renewable Energy Explained." https://www.eia.gov/energyexplained/renewable-sources/.

"Environmental Justice." n.d. "New York State Department of Environmental Conservation." http://www.dec.ny.gov/public/333.html.

Environmental Protection Agency. 2015. "What is Risk Assessment?"

Fahnestock, J. 1999. *Rhetorical Figures in Science.* New York: Oxford University Press.

Fahnestock, J., & Secor, M. 1985. "Toward a Modern Version of Stasis." In *Oldspeak/Newspeak,* edited by Charles W. Kneupper, 217–226. Arlington, TX: Rhetoric Society of America.

Fairclough, Norman. 1989. *Language and Power.* New York: Routledge.

Fairclough, Norman. 2008. *Analyzing Discourse: Textual Analysis for Social Research.* London: Routledge.

Fairclough, Norman, & Fairclough, I. 2015. To Frack or Not to Frack, That is the Question: "The Decision Against Exploratory Drilling in Lancashire as a Case of Deliberation in Institutional Contexts." http://wp.lancs.ac.uk/cperc-conf/files/2015/08/Isabela-and-Norman-Fairclough-CPE-of-Fracking-2015.pdf.

Feindt, Peter, & Oels, A. 2005. "Does Discourse Matter? Discourse Analysis in Environmental Policy Planning." *Journal of Environmental Policy and Planning,* 7(3), 161–173.

Finewood, Michael, & Stroup, L. J. 2012. "Fracking and the Neoliberalization of the Hydro-social Cycle in Pennsylvania's Marcellus Shale." *Journal of Contemporary Water Research & Education,* 147(1), 72–79.

Fiorino, Daniel. 1989. "Technical and Democratic Values in Risk Analysis." *Risk Analysis,* 9(3), 293–299.

Fiorino, Daniel. 1990. "Citizen Participation and Environmental Risk: A Survey of Institutional Mechanisms." *Science, Technology, & Human Values,* 15(2), 226–243.

Fischer, Frank. 1998. "Beyond Empiricism: Policy Inquiry in Postpostivist Perspective." *Policy Studies Journal,* 26(1), 129–146.

Fischer, Frank. 2000. *Citizens, Experts, and the Environment: The Politics of Local Knowledge.* Durham, NC: Duke University Press.

Fletcher, Robert. 2010. "Neoliberal Environmentality: Towards a Poststructuralist Policy Ecology of the Conservation Debate." *Conservation & Society,* 8(3), 171–181.

Fossil Fuel CO_2 Emissions by Nation. 2017. http://cdiac.ornl.gov/trends/emis/meth_reg.html.

Fuller, Sara, & McCauley, D. 2016. "Framing energy justice: Perspectives from Activism and Advocacy." *Energy Research and Social Justice*, 11, 1–8.

Funtowicz, Silvio, & Ravetz, J. R. 1993. "Science for the Post-normal Age." *Futures*, 25(7), 739–755.

Gehrke, Pat. 2014. "Ecological Validity and the Study of Publics: The Case for Organic Public Engagement Methods." *Public Understanding of Science*, 23(1), 77–91.

Geisler, Cheryl. 2003. *Analyzing Streams of Language: Twelve Steps to the Systemic Coding of Text, Talk and Other Verbal Data*. London: Longman.

George, Barbara. 2016a. "Environmental Justice and Precaution: Reimagining Public Risk Participation." *Reflections: Public Rhetoric, Civic Writing and Service Learning*, 16(1), 96–103.

George, Barbara. 2016b. "A Disability Studies Analysis of Rust Belt Narratives." *Disability and the Environment in American Literature*, edited by M. Cella, 151–172. Lanham, MD: Lexington.

George, Barbara. 2017a. "Ecological Journeys: From Higher Education to the Old Farm Trail." In *Narratives of Educating for Sustainability in Unsustainable Environments*, edited by Jane Haladay & Scott Hicks, 201–218. Lansing, MI: Michigan State University Press.

George, Barbara. 2017b. "Literacy, Praxis and Participation in Environmental Deliberation." In *Composing Feminist Interventions: Activism, engagement, praxis* edited by Kris Blair &d Lee Nickoson, 255–273. Fort Collins: WAC Clearinghouse.

George, Barbara. 2019a. "Communicating Activist Roles and Tools in Complex Energy Deliberation." *Communication Design Quarterly*, 7(1), 40–53. https://dl.acm.org/doi/10.1145/3331558.3331562.

George, Barbara. 2019b. "Language and Environmental Justice: Articulating Intersectionality within Energy Policy Deliberations". *Environmental Sociology*, 5(2), 149–162. https://www.tandfonline.com/doi/full/10.1080/23251042.2019.1605958.

Goggin, Peter. 2009. *Rhetorics, Literacies, and Narratives of Sustainability*. New York: Routledge.

Grabill, Jeffrey. 2001. *Community Literacy Programs and the Politics of Change*. New York: State University of New York Press.

Grabill, Jeffrey. 2007. *Writing Community Change: Designing Technologies for Citizen Action*. New York: Hampton Press.

Grabill, Jeffrey, & Simmons, M. 1998. "Towards a Civic Rhetoric for Technologically and Scientifically Complex Places: Invention, Performance and Participation." *Technical Communications Quarterly*, 7(4), 415–441.

Great Lakes Restoration Initiative. n.d. https://www.glri.us/.

Hajer, M. A. 1995. *The Politics of Environmental Discourse*. Oxford: Oxford University Press.

Hajer, M. A., & Versteeg, W.B. 2005. "A Decade of Discourse Analysis of Environmental Politics: Achievements, Challenges and Perspectives." *Journal of Environmental Policy and Planning*, 7(3), 175–184.

Halliday, M. A. K. 1978. *Language as Social Semiotic: The Social Interpretation of Language and Meaning*. Baltimore: University Park Press.

Haraway, Donna. 1996. "Situated Knowledges: The Science Question in Feminism and the Privilege of a Partial Perspective." In *Feminism and Science,* edited by Evelyn Fox Keller & Helen E. Longino, 249–263). New York: Oxford.

Harding, S. 1996. "Rethinking Standpoint Epistemology: What is "Strong Objectivity?" In *Feminism and Science,* edited by Evelyn Fox Keller and Helen E. Longino, 235–248. New York: Oxford.

Hardy, Charles. 2012. "Using the Environmental History of the Commonwealth to Enhance Pennsylvania and U.S. History Courses." *Pennsylvania History: A Journal of Mid-Atlantic Studies,* 79(4), 473–494.

Harré, Jens, Brockmeier, P., & Mühlhäusler, R. 1999. *Greenspeak: A Study of Environmental Discourse.* London: SAGE.

Harvey, D. 1999. "The Environment of Justice." In *Living with Nature: Environmental Politics as Cultural Discourse,* edited by F. Fischer & M. A. Hajer, 153–185. Oxford: Oxford University Press.

Heikkila, Tanya, Pierce, J. J., Gallaher, S., Kagan, J., Crow, D., & Weible, C. 2014. "Understanding a Period of Policy Change: The Case of Hydraulic Fracturing in Disclosure Policy in Colorado." *Review of Policy Research*, 31(2), 65–87.

Herndl, Carl G. & Brown, S. 1996. *Green Culture: Environmental Rhetoric in Contemporary America.* Madison: University of Wisconsin Press.

Herndl, Carl G., & Cutlip, L. L. 2013. "How Can We Act? A Praxiographical Program for the Rhetoric of Technology, Science, and Medicine." *Poroi,* 9(1), 1–13.

Holborow, Marnie. 2006. "Putting the Social Back into Language: Marx, Vološinov and Vygotsky Reexamined." *Studies In Language and Capitalism*, 1, 1–28.

Holifield, Ryan, Porter, M., & Walker, G. 2010. *Spaces of Environmental Justice.* Malden, MA: Wiley-Blackwell.

Hourdequin, Marion, Landres, P., Hanson, M., & Craig, D. 2012. "Ethical Implications of Democratic Theory for US Public Participation in Environmental Impact Assessment." *Environmental Impact Assessment Review,* 35, 37–44.

Hoyt, Kristopher. 2012. *Changing the Climate While Reproducing Power? Examining the Social Construction of "Renewable" Frames in Mass Print News Media 2000–2010* (Dissertation). University of Colorado.

Hurdle, J. 2015. "Report Revives Debate over Risks of Radiation from Drilling Waste." *State Impact.* https://stateimpact.npr.org/pennsylvania/2015/12/28/report-revives-debate-over-risks-of-radiation-from-drilling-waste/.

Hurdle, J. 2016. "EPA Bans Disposal of Fracking Waste Water at Public Treatment Plants." *State Impact.* https://stateimpact.npr.org/pennsylvania/2016/06/14/epa-bans-disposal-of-fracking-waste-water-at-public-treatment-plants/.

International Energy Agency. n.d. "Unconventional Oil." https://www.iea.org/about/faqs/oil/.

Isreal, Andrei., Wong-Paridi, G., Webler, T., & Stern, P. 2015. "Eliciting Public Concerns About an Emerging Energy Technology: The Case of Unconventional Shale Gas Development in the United States." *Energy Research and Social Justice* 8, 139–150.

Jalbert, Kirk. 2017. “Existing Water Monitoring Efforts.” Accessed February 1, 2017, https://www.fractracker.org/2017/02/susquehanna-river-basin-impacts-intro/.

Jasanoff, Sheila. 1987. “Contested Boundaries in Policy-Relevant Science.” *Social Studies of Science*, 17(2), 195–230.

Jasanoff, Sheila. 2003. “Technologies of Humility: Citizens Participation in Governing Science.” *Minerva,* 41(3), 223–244.

Jereczek, P. 2017. “Fracking in Dairy Country.” *FracTracker Alliance.* https://www.fractracker.org/2017/04/fracking-dairy-country/.

Journet, Debra. 2012. “Narrative Turns in Writing Studies Research.” In *Writing studies research in Practice: Methods and Methodologies,* edited by Lee Nickoson & Mary P. Sheridan, 13–24. Carbondale: Southern Illinois University Press.

Kear, Andrew. 2011. *Unconventional Politics of Unconventional Gas: Environmental Reframing and Policy Change* (Dissertation). Colorado State University.

Kear, Andrew, & Forbis, R. 2015. *Fractured Politics: Disparate Political Responses to Marcellus Shale Energy Development in Pennsylvania and New York.* Pocatello: Idaho State University.

Keller, Evylyn Fox, & Longino, H. E. (Eds.). 1996. *Feminism & Science.* New York: Oxford University Press.

Killingsworth, Jimmie, & Palmer, J. S. 1992. *Ecospeak; Rhetorics and Environmental Politics in America.* Carbondale: Southern Illinois University Press.

Kinchy, Abby, Parks, S., & Jalbert, K. 2016. “Fractured knowledge: Mapping the Gaps in Public and Private Water Monitoring Efforts in Areas Affected by Shale Gas Development.” *Environment and Planning C: Politics and Space,* 34(5), 879–899.

Klein, J. 2010. *Interdisciplinarity: History, Theory, and Practice.* Detroit: Wayne State University Press.

Kirk, Karen. 2023. “Yale Climate Connections. Which State is Winning at Renewable Energy Production?” https://yaleclimateconnections.org/2023/02/us-state-with-most-renewable-energy-production/.

Kowalski, K. 2014. “Fracking Wastewater is Big Business in Ohio.” *Midwest Energy News.* http://midwestenergynews.com/2014/07/18/fracking-wastewater-is-big-business-in-ohio/.

Kress, G. 2012. “Multimodal Discourse Analysis.” In *The Routledge handbook of discourse analysis,* edited by James Paul Gee & Michael Handford, 35–50. New York: Routledge.

Lafferty, Michael. (Ed.). 1979. *Ohio’s Natural Heritage.* Columbus: The Ohio Academy of Science.

Lakoff, George. 2010. “Why it Matters How We Frame the Environment.” *Environmental Communication,* 4(1), 70–81.

Lash, Scott, Szerszynski & Wynne. (Eds.). 1996. *Risk, Environment, & Modernity: Towards a New Ecology.* London: SAGE.

Lefsrud, L. M., & Meyer, R. E. 2012. “Science or Science Fiction? Professionals’ Discursive Constructions of Climate Change.” *Organization Studies,* 33(11), 1477–1506.

Lemke, Jay. 2012. "Multimedia and Discourse Analysis." In *The Routledge Handbook of Discourse Analysis,* edited by James Paul Gee & Michael Handford, 35–50. New York: Routledge.

List of the Harmed. 2017. *PA Alliance for Clean Water and Air.* https://pennsylvaniaallianceforcleanwaterandair.wordpress.com/the-list/.

Long, Eleanor. 2008. *Community Literacy and the Rhetoric of Local Publics.* Parlor Press, WAC Clearinghouse.

Long, Eleanor. 2009. "Rhetorical Techne, Local Knowledge, and Challenges in Contemporary Activism." In *Rhetorics, literacies, and Narratives of Sustainability,* edited by P. Goggin, 11–38. New York: Routledge.

Lovejoy, Kristen, & Saxton, G. D. 2012. "Information, Community, and Action: How Nonprofit Organizations use Social Media." *Journal of Computer-Mediated Communication,* 17(3), 337–353.

Lucas, Hugo, Carbajo, R., Machiba, T., Zhukov, E., & Cabeza, L. F. 2021. "Improving Public Attitude Towards Renewable Energy." *Energies.* https://doi.org/103390/en14154521.

Malin, Stephanie, & DeMaster, K. 2016. "A Devil's Bargain: Rural Environmental Injustices and Hydraulic Fracturing on Pennsylvania's Farms." *Journal of Rural Studies*, 47(A), 278–290.

May, Vivian. 2015. *Pursuing Intersectionality, Unsettling Dominant Imaginaries.* New York: Routledge.

McGreavy, Bridie, Silka, B., & Hart, D. 2012. "Creating a Place for Environmental Communication Research in Sustainability Science." *Environmental Communication,* 6(1), 23–43.

Moss, Pamela, & Falconer-Al Hendi, K. 2007. *Feminisms in Geography: Rethinking Space, Place, and Knowledges.* Lanham, MD: Rowman and Littlefield.

Murray, Jeff. 2017. "Crestwood Drops Seneca Lake Storage Plans." Accessed May 10, 2017. http://www.stargazette.com/story/news/2017/05/10/crestwood-drops-seneca-lake-natural-gas-storage-plans/316228001/

Myerson, George, & Ryden, Y. 1996. *The Language of the Environment: A New Rhetoric*. London: Routledge.

Nash, Roderick. 1968. *Wilderness and the American Mind.* New Haven, CT: Yale University Press.

New York State Department of Health. 2015. *A Public Review of High Volume Hydraulic Fracturing for Shale Gas Development.* https://www.health.ny.gov/press/reports/docs/high_volume_hydraulic_fracturing.pdf.

NYSERDA. 2023a. "Large Scale Renewables in Your Community." https://www.nyserda.ny.gov/All-Programs/Clean-Energy-Standard/Landowners-and-Local-Governments.

NYSERDA. 2023b. "Clean Energy Standard." https://www.nyserda.ny.gov/All-Programs/Clean-Energy-Standard.

NYSERDA. 2023c. "Clean Energy Siting Resources" https://www.nyserda.ny.gov/All-Programs/Clean-Energy-Siting-Resources.

Northeast Gas Association. n.d. "NGA Issue Brief, Marcellus Shale." http://www.northeastgas.org/marcellus_shale.php.

Nixon, Robert. 2011. *Slow Violence and the Environmentalism of the Poor*. Cambridge, MA: Harvard University Press.

ODNR Division of Forestry. n.d.. "History of Ohio State Forests." http://forestry.ohiodnr.gov/history.

Ogneva-Himmelberger, Y., & Yao, L. 2015. "Spatial Distribution of Unconventional Gas Wells and Human Populations in the Marcellus Region in the United States: Vulnerability Analysis." *Applied Geography*, 60, 165–174.

Ohio Department of Natural Resources. 2014. "Ohio Announces Tougher Permit Conditions for Drilling Activities Near Faults and Areas near Seismic Activity." Accessed April 11, 2014. http://ohiodnr.gov/news/post/ohio-announces-tougher-permit-conditions-for- drilling-activities-near-faults-and-areas-of-seismic-activit y.

Ohio Environmental Protection Agency. 2015. "Ohio EPA and Environmental Justice." http://ohioepa.custhelp.com/app/answers/detail/a_id/1097/~/ohio-epa-and-environmental-justice.

Ottinger, Gwen. 2012. "Changing Knowledge, Local Knowledge, and Knowledge Gaps: STS Insights into Procedural Justice." *Science, Technology, & Human Values,* 38(2), 250–270.

Olson-Hazboun, Shawn, Howe, P., & Leiserowitz, A. 2018. "The Influence of Extractive Activities on Public Support for Renewable Energy Policy." *Energy Policy*, 123, 117–126.

Oullette, J. 2017. "The Viability of Digital Spaces as Sites for Transnational Feminist Engagement." In *Composing Feminist Interventions: Activism, Engagement, Praxis,* edited by Kris Blair & Lee Nickoson, 275–296. Fort Collins: WAC Clearinghouse.

Pennsylvania Department of Environmental Protection. n.d. Office of Environmental Justice. http://www.dep.pa.gov/publicparticipation/officeofenvironmentaljustice/pages/default.aspx.

Philips, S. 2016. "Federal Public Health Report Highlight Contaminants in Dimock's Water." *State Impact.* https://stateimpact.npr.org/pennsylvania/2016/05/25/federal-public-health-report-highlights-contaminants-in-dimocks-water/.

Reed, Mark. 2008. "Stakeholder Participation for Environmental Management: A Literature Review." *Biological Conservation,* 141(10), 2417–2431.

Reed, Mark, Graves, A., Dandy, N., Posthumus, H., Hubacek, K., Morris,…Stringer, L. 2009. "Whose In and Why? A Typology of Stakeholder Analysis Methods for Natural Resource Management." *Journal of Environmental Management,* 90(5), 1933–1949.

ReImagine Appalachia. 2024. *About Us*. Retrieved from https://reimagineappalachia.org/about/.

Rowe, Gene, & Frewer, L. J. 2004. "Evaluating Public-Participation Exercises: a Research Agenda." *Science, Technology, & Human Values,* 29(4), 512–556.

Rowe, Gene, & Frewer, L. G. 2005. "A Typology of Public Engagement Mechanisms." *Science, Technology, & Human Values,* 30(2), 251–290.

Royster, Jacqueline, & Kirsch, G. 2012. *Feminist Rhetorical Practices: New Horizons for Rhetoric, Composition, and Literacy Studies.* Carbondale, IL: Southern Illinois University Press.

Sauer, Beverly. 2003. *The Rhetoric of Risk: Technical Documentation in Hazardous Environments*. Mahwah, NJ: Erlbaum.

Schippa, Edward. 1998. "Constructing Reality through Definitions: The Politics of Meaning." *The Center for Interdisciplinary Studies of Writing*. Minneapolis: University of Minnesota.

Schiappa, Edward. 2003. *Defining Reality: Definitions and Politics of Meaning*. Carbondale: Southern Illinois University Press.

Schiappa, J. 2017. "Assessing Intersectional Activism Through a Comparison of Two Slutwalks." In *Composing feminist Interventions: Activism, Engagement, Praxis*, edited by Kris Blair & Lee Nickoson, 297–316. Fort Collins: WAC Clearinghouse.

Schirrmeister, Mira. 2014. "Controversial Futures – Discourse Analysis on Utilizing the 'Fracking' Technology in Germany." *European Journal of Futures Research*, 2(38). https://eujournalfuturesresearch.springeropen.com/articles/10.1007/s40309-014-0038-5.

Scholz, Roland W. 2011. *Environmental Literacy in Science and Society: from Knowledge to Decisions*. New York: Cambridge University Press.

Selfe, Cynthia, & Hawisher, G. 2012. "Exceeding the Bounds of the Interview: Feminism, Mediation, Narrative, and Conversations about Digital Literacy." In *Writing Studies Research in Practice: Methods and Methodologies*, edited by Lee Nickoson & Mary P. Sheridan, 36–52. Carbondale: Southern Illinois University Press.

Shalefield Stories: A Project of Friends of the Harmed. n.d. http://www.shalefieldstories.org/.

Simmons, Michele. 2007. *Participation and Power: Civic Discourse in Environmental Policy Decisions*. Albany: State University of New York Press.

Simmons, Michele, & Grabill, J. 2007. "Toward a Civic rhetoric for Technologically and Scientifically Complex Places: Invention, Performance, and Participation." *NCTE*, 58(3), 419–448.

Sisson, M. 2012. "Stinchcomb Memorial." *Cleveland Historical*, accessed November 10, 2017. https://clevelandhistorical.org/items/show/388.

Smooth, Wendy. 2013. "Intersectionality from Theoretical Framework to Policy Intervention." In *Situating intersectionality: Politics, Policy, and Power*, edited by Angelina Wilson, 11–41. New York: Palgrave Macmillan.

Southwest Pennsylvania Environmental Health Project. 2021. http://www.environmentalhealthproject.org/.

Southwest Pennsylvania Environmental Health Project. 2021. Air quality. http://www.environmentalhealthproject.org/.

Southwest Pennsylvania Environmental Health Project. 2021. Health issues. http://www.environmentalhealthproject.org/.

Späth, Philip, & Rohracher, H. 2010. "Energy Regions: The Transformative Power of Regional Discourses on Socio-Technical Futures." *Research Policy*, 39(1), 449–458.

Steffek, Jens. 2009. "Discursive Legitimation in Environmental Governance." *Forest Policy and Economics*, 11, 313–318.

Steingraber, Sandra. 1997. *Living Downstream: A Scientist's Personal Investigation of Cancer and the Environment*. New York: Vintage.

Steinzor, N., & Baizel, B. 2015. "Wasting Away: Four States' Failure to Manage Oil and Gas Waste from the Marcellus and Utica Shale." *Earthworks.* https://www.earthworksaction.org/files/publications/WastingAway-FINAL-lowres.pdf.

Stephens, Jennie, C., Rand, G., & Melneck, L. 2009. "Wind Energy in U.S. Media: A Comparative State-level Analysis of a Critical Climate Change." *Mitigation Technical Environmental Communication,* 3(2), 168–190.

Stibbe, Arran. 2015. *Ecolinguistics: Language, Ecology, and the Stories We Live By.* New York: Routledge.

Stradling, David. 2010. *The Nature of New York: An Environmental History of the Empire State.* Ithaca: Cornell University Press.

Stradling, David, & Stradling, R. 2008. "Perceptions of the Burning River: Deindustrialization and Cleveland's Cuyahoga River." *Environmental History,* 13(3), 515–535.

Sullivan, Patricia. 2003. "Feminism and Methodology in Composition Studies." In *Feminism and Composition: A Critical Sourcebook,* edited by Gesa E. Kirsch, Faye Spencer Maor, Lance Massey, Lee Nickoson-Massey, & Mary P. Sheridan-Rabideau, 124–139. Urbana: Bedford/St. Martin's.

Szerszynski, B. 1996. "On Knowing What to do: Environmentalism and the Modern Problematic." In *Risk, Environment, & Modernity: Towards a New Ecology,* edited by Scott Lash, Bronislaw Szerszynski, & Brian Wynne, 104–138. London: Sage.

Tarr, Joel. 1999. "The Environmental History of Pennsylvania. Pennsylvania History." *A Journal of Mid-Atlantic Studies,* 66(4), 445–447.

U.S. Department of Energy. 2015. *Fossil Fuel/Conventional Fuel.*

USDA Forest Service. 2017. "Forest Inventory and Analysis National Program." Accessed May 31, 2017. https://www.fia.fs.fed.us/.

USGS. 2016. "What is Hydraulic Fracturing?" Accessed November 16, 2016. https://www2.usgs.gov/faq/categories/10132/3814.

Van Dijk, Teun. 2003. "Critical Discourse Analysis." In *The Handbook of Discourse Analysis,* edited by D. Schriffrin, D. Tannen, & H. Hamilton, 349–371. New Jersey: Wiley-Blackwell.

Van Leeuwen, Theodore. 2007. "Legitimation in Discourse and Communication." *Discourse & Communication,* 1(1), 91–112.

Wajcman, Judy. 2007. "From Women and Technology to Gendered Technoscience." *Information, Communication & Society,* 10(3), 287–298.

Walker, Gordon. 2010. "Environmental Justice, Impact Assessment and the Politics of Knowledge: The Implications of Assessing the Social Distribution of Environmental Outcomes." *Environmental Impact Assessment Review,* 30(5), 312–318.

Warren, Karen. 2000. *Ecofeminist Philosophy: A Western perspective on What It Is and Why it Matters.* Lanham, MD: Rowman and Littlefield.

We Are Seneca Lake. 2016. "Seneca Lake Defenders." http://www.wearesenecalake.com/seneca-lake-defendes/.

"What is a Cracker and Why Should I Care?" 2017. *AFPM.* http://education.afpm.org/petrochemicals/what-is-a-cracker-and-why-should-i-care/.

Whiteside, Karen. 2006. *Precautionary Politics.* Cambridge, MA: Routledge.

Whyte, A., & Burton, I. (Eds.). 1980. *Environmental Risk Assessment*. New York: Scientific Committee on Problems of the Environment.

Wodak, Ruth, & Meyer, M. (Eds.). 2009. "Critical Discourse Analysis: History, Agenda, Theory and Methodology." *Methods of Critical Discourse Analysis,* 1–33. London: Sage.

Woehrle, Lynne. 2014. "Intersectionality and Social Change." In *Intersectionality and Social Change: Research in Social Movements, Conflicts and Change,* edited by L. Whoerle, 1–20. Bingley: Emerald Group.

Woodall, Candy. 2016. "PA Supreme Court says ACT 13 Gave Oil and Gas Industry Special Treatment, Violated Constitution." Accessed September 28, 2016. http://www.pennlive.com/news/2016/09/pa_supreme_court_says_act_13_g.html.

Yeoman, Barry. 2014. "Lake Erie Deathwatch." Accessed August 2014. http://archive.onearth.org/article/lake-erie-death-watch.

Young, Iris. 1990. *Democracy and Inclusion.* Cambridge: Oxford University Press.

Index

About the Author

Barbara George is a teacher and researcher in environmental communication, technical writing, and within writing studies pedagogy at Carnegie Mellon University.

Barbara's research focuses on linguistic explorations of the intersections of environmental risk and communication, issues of intersectionality within environmental deliberation, and environmental justice within environmental communication. Additionally, Barbara explores the use of narrative in finding new ways to "reimagine" environmental frames, particularly in Rust Belt communities. Barbara's work appears in *Composition Forum*, *Environmental Sociology*, and *Communication Design Quarterly* among others.

www.ingramcontent.com/pod-product-compliance
Ingram Content Group UK Ltd.
Pitfield, Milton Keynes, MK11 3LW, UK
UKHW041839031026
15587UKWH00002B/874

9 781666 926484